Sleep Paralysis

D1554764

Sleep Paralysis

Night-mares, Nocebos, and the Mind-Body Connection

SHELLEY R. ADLER

RUTGERS UNIVERSITY PRESS

NEW BRUNSWICK, NEW JERSEY, AND LONDON

LIBRARY OF CONGRESS CATALOGING-IN-PUBLICATION DATA

Adler, Shelley R., 1963–
    Sleep paralysis : night-mares, nocebos, and the mind-body connection / Shelley R. Adler.
      p. cm.
Includes bibliographical references and index.
    ISBN 978–0–8135–4885–2 (hardcover : alk. paper) — ISBN 978–0–8135–4886–9 (pbk. : alk. paper)
    I. Nightmares.   2. Sleep disorders.   3. Mind and body.   I. Title.
BF1099.N53A44   2011
154.6—dc22   2010004654

A British Cataloging-in-Publication record for this book is available from the British Library.

Visit our Web site: http://rutgerspress.rutgers.edu

Manufactured in the United States of America

For Nancy, Sarah, Kate, Jeffrey, and Scott
In memory of my mother, Shoshana Adler

CONTENTS

ACKNOWLEDGMENTS

This book has been a long-term labor of love, and many people have helped to sustain my efforts. I am grateful to Michael Owen Jones, Carole Browner, and the late Alan Dundes and Donald Ward for their inspiration and support. David Hufford and Allan Cheyne have been tremendously generous, and their ground-breaking sleep paralysis scholarship has been foundational in my own work. I want to thank Susan Folkman, Kevin Grumbach, Ellen Hughes, and Helen Loeser for their apparently limitless wisdom and encouragement concerning this project. Conversations with colleagues at the Osher Center for Integrative Medicine have been invaluable—and the inspired perfectionism of Rick Scott's and Yvette Coulter's bibliographic and technical expertise, as well as scholarly detective work, have made managing the details a pleasure.

The writing of this book was supported by Grant #G13 LM008224 from the National Library of Medicine (National Institutes of Health). My mind-body research has also been sustained through my role as director of education at the UCSF Osher Center for Integrative Medicine, with the support of an endowed chair from the Osher Foundation. This position has afforded me many opportunities to share my nocebo work with health professional students, residents, and faculty—and to learn much from our discussions.

Mac Marshall, Studies in Medical Anthropology series editor, has been a steady source of inspiration, guidance, and enthusiasm. I would also like to thank Adi Hovav and Doreen Valentine, editors; Marlie Wasserman, director; and Marilyn Campbell and Jamie Greene, prepress, at Rutgers University Press for making the publication process such a pleasure.

Kazumi Honda, Katherine Hillman, Maya Jairam, and Sean Clarke con-tributed the illustrations that greatly enhance the depictions of night-mares in this book. Thank you for your generosity.

I am grateful for the support of friends and my extended family, who have helped me in so many ways, from faithfully clipping relevant newspaper articles to offering me writing space (both figuratively and literally) while they enter-tained our children. My heartfelt thanks to Kathleen Kerr; Carole and Robert Millhauser; Scott, Richard, and Mark Showen; and the B-team: Peter, Lauren, and Becky. Thanks, also, to the friends who enthusiastically embraced this book's topic (and agreed to be interviewed) during the early years of the project: Dorrie Nussenbaum, Anath Ranon, and Chris Cassady.

I am deeply indebted to all of the people who trusted me with retellings of their night-mares, but, most of all, to the Hmong men and women who openheartedly shared the challenges of their immigrant experiences, as well as their joys. *Ua tsaug ntau.*

Above all, I thank Nancy—and Scott, Jeffrey, Kate, and Sarah—for their support, enthusiasm, and good humor. In the introduction to John Waller's 1816 essay on the night-mare, he writes: "The enjoyment of comfortable and undisturbed sleep is certainly to be ranked among the greatest blessings which heaven has bestowed upon mankind." It is a testament to the youthful exuberance of my four wonderful children that, despite my writing into the wee hours about the most loathsome and terrifying nocturnal demons, I was sufficiently exhausted to sleep soundly each night.

Sweet dreams—

SRA

San Francisco, California

Sleep Paralysis

Introduction

On a winter morning in early January 1981, Xiong Tou Xiong, a twenty-nine-year-old man, was found dead in the bed of his Portland, Oregon home. He had not been ill; his death was sudden and unexpected. Two days later, Yong Leng Thao, a forty-seven-year-old man, died on the way to a Portland hospital after his wife found him lying in his bed, unresponsive (Davidson 1981). He had been up late watching television with an uncle and had gone to bed after midnight, briefly waking his wife. Both were soon asleep. "Then came his labored breathing, so loud that it awakened her. She shook him. . . . [In the] next moments of horror, she realized that she could do nothing more" (Curry 1981, B16).

Both of the men who died were Laotian Hmong refugees who had recently immigrated to the United States. Their deaths were brought to the attention of Larry Lewman, the medical examiner of Multnomah County. In reviewing recent reports, Lewman soon found two additional cases of sudden, unexpected death. Searching for further clues, he telephoned the coroner's office in St. Paul, Minnesota, a city in which, like Portland, many Southeast Asian refugees had settled. As forensic scientist Michael McGee recalls, he was told: "We have a large Southeast Asian population here, and we can't figure out what's happening. We have no idea why these people are dying. Would there be any chance you guys are experiencing the same thing?" (Meier 2004).

In fact, death records in St. Paul showed that four Laotian Hmong refugees had died suddenly in their sleep. A mysterious pattern was beginning to emerge: all of the victims had died unexpectedly; all were men between the ages of twenty-five and fifty; all were apparently healthy; and all had died while they were asleep. Also, in all cases for which autopsies had been conducted,[1] findings were negative.

Sudden deaths among the Hmong continued throughout the mid-1980s, but no medical cause could be found. In 1986, when I first learned of the

1

unexplained nocturnal deaths, I was a graduate student in Los Angeles, studying traditional belief narratives. What little I had heard about the syndrome—that seemingly healthy people died in the night, on their backs, with looks of terror on their faces—was strangely evocative of the traditional nocturnal pressing spirit attacks I had been researching. I knew that these nocturnal visitations (termed "sleep paralysis" in the scientific literature) were characterized as terrifying, *but ultimately harmless* experiences. Still, as I continued to research the nocturnal spirit attacks in different sociocultural contexts, I became intrigued by the possibility of a relationship between the traditional nocturnal experiences and the Hmong immigrants' sudden deaths.

I began to study the pattern of the unexplained fatalities and learned that the first reported case of what would later become known as Sudden Unexpected Nocturnal Death Syndrome (SUNDS) had actually occurred in 1977, with the death of Ly Doua in Orange County, California (Maxwell 1981a, 1981b). The incidence of the deaths peaked in 1981 and 1982, and it was this preponderance of cases that resulted in the recognition of a pattern that might not otherwise have been noticed until much later. The median age at death for victims of the syndrome was thirty-three, and the median length of time that they had been living in the United States before death was seventeen months.

What was most striking for me, as a student of traditional narrative, however, was the fact that the symptoms of SUNDS-related events reported by epidemiologists mirrored the characteristics of the nocturnal pressing spirit attack as it has been known in folk tradition across cultures and throughout history: the victim's impression of wakefulness, inability to move or speak, realistic perception of the immediate environment, intense fear and anxiety, lying in a supine position, feeling pressure on the chest, difficulty breathing, and awareness of a "presence" that is often seen or heard. The *night-mare,* as I have chosen to call this encounter (for lack of a contemporary, widely recognized term), is distinct from all other sleep phenomena, including generic "bad dreams" and night terrors. The prevalence of the night-mare is remarkably high, with 25–30 percent of healthy people around the world experiencing at least one episode. In the United States, though, the night-mare leads a paradoxical existence: the experience is simultaneously very common and little known.

Across cultures and throughout history, encounters with nocturnal pressing spirits have many similarities. Although these commonalities seem to point to a shared biological framework, individual experiences can also contain distinctive details that prompt local, cultural interpretations. The night-mare experience, therefore, presents a unique opportunity to study the reciprocal influence of culture and biology by providing a lens through which to view the interconnectedness of mind and body (Hinton, Hufford, and Kirmayer 2005); the night-mare illustrates the dynamics and consequences of the interaction between cultural beliefs and human physiology.

Before venturing further, it is worth noting the lexical challenge at the heart of this inquiry into such a common, yet unfamiliar, experience. Contemporary English terminology is inadequate in its ability to reference "an encounter with a nocturnal pressing spirit"—there is literally no word to describe the experience. One solution to this dearth of vocabulary would be to adopt the name of a culture-specific spirit to represent the experience globally; for example, by using Newfoundland's *Old Hag* to refer to all nocturnal pressing spirit encounters. This strategy, though, conflates local representations with broader understandings. On the other hand, selecting a term such as *sleep paralysis* might seem to imply that I am privileging the scientific explanation as the "true" account of the event. In the end, after choosing from a number of poor candidates, I am left with the (perhaps inelegant but) historically potent *night-mare* to denote the experience.

I use the term *night-mare*—with a hyphen—in its original sense of a nocturnal visit of an evil being that threatens to press the very life out of its terrified victim. The *Oxford English Dictionary* (1989) defines this creature as "a spirit or monster supposed to beset people . . . by night, settling upon them when they are asleep and producing a feeling of suffocation by its weight." In the field of sleep research, this experience is termed "sleep paralysis": an individual, in the process of falling asleep or awakening, finds himself or herself completely awake, but unable to move or speak. The person often feels an oppressive weight on the chest or body and a sense of suffocation. Frequently, he or she sees a shadowy or indistinct shape approaching and becomes increasingly terrified. The episode may last from seconds to minutes, until the "sleeper" is suddenly released and able to move once more. Sleep researchers understand these sensations to be a disturbance of the normal regulation of sleep, in which the muscular paralysis characteristic of REM sleep—and designed to keep us from acting out our dreams—occurs during a state of waking awareness (Hinton, Hufford, and Kirmayer 2005).

Further complicating the issue of nomenclature are two sleep occurrences that are seemingly related to, but actually quite distinct from, the night-mare. One of these nocturnal events is commonly referred to as a "nightmare" (without the hyphen) and indicates a frightening dream. Although, as we shall see, the etymology of the word *nightmare* is closely connected to sleep paralysis; in contemporary use, the term refers broadly to any disturbing dream. In a typical bad dream, the sleeper awakens in the middle of a sleep cycle and experiences a strong, unpleasant emotional response, as well as vivid (if often short-term) recall of the features of the dream. This standard anxiety dream, although it can be extremely distressing, is unrelated to the night-mare encounter in both its symptoms and the specific stage of sleep in which it appears (Hufford 1976, 1982; Liddon 1967).

The other sleep event that is often mistakenly merged with the night-mare—because of our inadequate terminology—is the "night terror," or *pavor nocturnus*. During a night terror, the sleeper seems to awaken in fear and agitation, screaming and thrashing about, but then falls back asleep and remembers little or nothing of the incident in the morning (Kryger, Roth, and Dement 2000).[2] Both generic bad dreams and night terrors have been confused with sleep paralysis in medical and early sleep literature—but, significantly, never by those who have experienced a night-mare attack.

In relying on a mere hyphen to distinguish such an impactful experience (night-mare versus bad dream), I am reminded of a passage from anthropologists Nancy Scheper-Hughes and Margaret Lock's seminal work, "The Mindful Body: A Prolegomenon to Future Medical Anthropological Research," in which they explain the difficulty of describing a phenomenon that is not accompanied by accurate terminology:

> As both medical anthropologists and clinicians struggle to view humans and the experience of illness and suffering from an integrated perspective, they often find themselves trapped by the Cartesian legacy. We lack a precise vocabulary with which to deal with mind-body-society interactions and so are left suspended in hyphens, testifying to the disconnect of our thoughts. We are forced to resort to such fragmented concepts as the bio-social, the psycho-somatic, the somato-social as altogether feeble ways of expressing the myriad ways in which the mind speaks through the body, and the ways in which society is inscribed on the expectant canvas of human flesh. (1987, 10)

The challenge Scheper-Hughes and Lock describe not only resonates with my own struggle to locate a "precise vocabulary," but also points to the fractured concept of mind-body that complicates any discussion of the night-mare. One of the assumptions that has been paradigmatic to biomedicine and that shapes so much of scientific thought more broadly is the much-noted Cartesian dualism that separates the body from the mind and the real (visible, measurable, evidence based) from the unreal (supernatural, religious, unprovable). This dichotomy, however, is a culturally and historically specific construction that is not universally shared. In order to begin to understand the night-mare phenomenon as it has been and is currently experienced by so many people worldwide, we must start by suspending "our usual belief and cultural commitment to the mind/body, seen/unseen, natural/supernatural, magical/rational, rational/irrational, and real/unreal oppositions and assumptions" (Scheper-Hughes and Lock 1987, 6). It is neither necessary nor advisable (nor indeed possible) to dispense with these notions permanently, but it is essential to adopt a wider lens in order to view the complexity of this phenomenon more completely. The medical folklorist David J. Hufford justifies the need for this inclusive, holistic approach:

> Analyses that "fully explain" local traditions by either psychosocial etiology or as "cultural frosting on a biological cake," do implicitly contradict local beliefs, showing them to be fundamentally incorrect accounts of

reality. This interpretation may sometimes be the most plausible one, but exclusionist approaches make such reductive conclusions the starting points rather than hypotheses to be empirically tested. (1988, 510)

Beginning with the assumption that human beings are simultaneously biological and cultural, my challenge is to present a balanced approach—one that avoids initially privileging either biology (bodily states or processes) or traditional belief (mind or mental processes). Anthropologist Daniel Moerman provides a useful framework for this strategy with his notion of the *meaning response*, "the psychological and physiological effects of meaning in the treatment of illness" (2002, 14). When the meaning effects comprise positive outcomes, they include what is often referred to as the "placebo effect"; when the outcomes are negative, they include what has been termed the "nocebo effect."

Placebo comes from the Latin word meaning "I shall please." The Catholic Vespers of the Office of the Dead began with the word *placebo* (*Placebo Dominum in regione vivorum*), and, in the thirteenth century, the term was adopted as the name of that service. Because some people attended the funeral service and sang the Placebo (that is, simulated mourning) hoping to be rewarded by the relatives of the deceased, the word came to mean "a sycophant." It is in this sense that Chaucer, writing in the fourteenth century, observed: "Flatterers are the Devil's chaplain, always singing *Placebo*" (c. 1390).[3] At the end of the eighteenth century, the word began to be applied to sham medical substances (simulated treatments) that physicians knowingly doled out to "please" patients (even though the treatments occasionally had positive effects). In the early nineteenth century, a medical dictionary defined *placebo* as "an epithet given to any medicine adapted more to please than benefit the patient" (Hooper 1811, 942). Over the next 150 years, *placebo* transformed in meaning from an inert substance given deliberately to please a patient into a treatment believed efficacious by a physician and later determined to be inert (Harrington 2008). Today, placebos are increasingly studied as keys to the mysteries of the beneficial (and often unplanned and unanticipated) effects that occur in the process of treating disease. As a simple example, an often-cited instance of the positive effects of the meaning response is found in the study of a suburban Pennsylvania hospital that showed that surgical patients who stayed in a hospital room with a window view of a natural setting recovered more quickly than a matched sample of patients who had a view of a brick wall (Ulrich 1984).

In contrast to the positive effect of the meaning response, the *nocebo* (from the Latin for "I shall harm") phenomenon consists of a negative outcome. An example of "placebo's evil twin" is found in the results of a large study conducted by sociologist David P. Phillips and colleagues that examined the cause of death of adult Chinese Americans and randomly selected matched European American controls. The researchers found that "Chinese Americans, but not whites, die significantly earlier" than expected "if they have a combination of disease and birth year which Chinese astrology and medicine considers ill-fated" (Phillips, Ruth, and Wagner 1993, 1142). For example, among Chinese Americans who died of illnesses related to lung diseases (such as bronchitis, emphysema, and asthma), those who were born in *metal* years"—lungs are the organ of metal (Beinfield and Korngold 1991)—had an average age at death that was five years younger than among those born in other years who also died from these lung diseases. No such differences were evident in a large series of white European Americans who died of similar causes in the same period. Furthermore, the intensity of the effect was shown to be correlated with "the strength of commitment to traditional Chinese culture." According to Moerman, it is clear from this case that the significant difference in longevity "among Chinese Americans (up to 6 or 7% of length of life) is not due to having Chinese genes, but to having Chinese ideas, to knowing the world in Chinese ways" (2002, 78). The beliefs people hold and the ways in which men and women understand the world and their place in it can have profound consequences for their health.

Many people find it enormously difficult to accept the possibility of any sociocultural or psychological influence on illnesses that appear to be obviously biological or physiological. I have taught medical students and residents at an academic medical center for many years, and I can attest to the fact that it is still the case that much standard health professional training teaches that diseases are either wholly organic or wholly psychological—and that it is crucial to distinguish sharply between the two. As anthropologist Robert Hahn notes, "the fact is that phenomena that essentially come down to what people believe are conceptually difficult in our medical system" (as well as, I would add, in the medical social sciences). "Health is thought to be a biological phenomenon. More psychosomatic elements are hard to deal with" (Reid 2002, HE-01).

We know that understandings of the specific "facts" of health and illness differ dramatically in medical cultures around the world. How the proper sick role is understood, appropriate relationships between patient and healer defined, or causes of disease explained, varies widely. Even with the universalist biomedical system, illness (and also health) has distinct meanings in different places. In these diverse contexts, in which

> meaning shapes so much of life, it is not surprising that meaning also influences the effectiveness of medical treatment. There is more to biology than biology. This isn't always the case (leaping from a sixteenth-story window ledge will not be much affected by desire, will, or culture). But far more often than we realize, what appears to be an "obvious" biological matter is richly freighted with meaning, history, tradition, or the like; or requires consciousness to do its thing. Indeed, it is probably wise to assume this is the case until it's proven otherwise. (Moerman 2002, 702)

The night-mare, poised as it is between the supernatural and natural worlds, and between the meaningful and the biological, is perfectly positioned to teach us about the seamless connection between our minds and our bodies.

I have conducted field and archival research on the experience and interpretation of the night-mare assault over the past twenty years. In the course of this work, I have studied cultural, historical, and scientific explanations of the night-mare; analyzed hundreds of interviews I conducted with night-mare sufferers, sleep researchers, physicians, historians, museum curators, and others; and examined thousands of postings on Internet listservs, Web logs, and video-sharing Web sites by people who have experienced sleep paralysis. This book traces the trajectory of my own inquiry into the night-mare, from the experience's remarkable cross-cultural consistency and historical continuity; to perspectives on the phenomenon from psychology, biomedicine, and sleep research; to an in-depth look at the Hmong night-mare; and ends with an illustration of the nocebo-linked interplay between meaning (mind) and biology (body).

1

Consistencies

Cross-cultural Patterns

I lay me down to sleep;
No night-mare shall plague me
Until they swim all the waters that flow upon the earth
And count all the stars that shine in the sky.

—German charm against night-mares (Kuhn 1859)

Imagine feeling very tired, going to bed, and quickly falling asleep. Your rest is soon disturbed, though, by some sort of rustling noise. You open your eyes and recognize the normal features of your bedroom in the shadowy darkness, but, when you try to sit up, you realize that you are paralyzed; you are unable to move your arms or legs, or even turn your head. With sudden, sickening dread and overwhelming terror, you sense an evil presence approaching. You struggle and try to scream for help, but you still cannot move or make a sound. The sinister being looms over you for a moment, then climbs onto your bed and settles heavily on your chest, crushing the breath out of you.

This experience is the night-mare[1] and its key features are the same the world over: knowing that you are awake, perceiving your surroundings realistically, being unable to move, feeling overwhelmed by intense terror and anxiety, sensing an evil presence, feeling crushing pressure on your chest, trying desperately to breathe, and lying helplessly on your back. These elements are easy to identify in the following account:

I am 52 years old. My [night-mares] started in my mid 20s. I remember the first time it happened. I had a new baby and was napping in the afternoon because I also worked in the evenings. Suddenly, I was wide awake except for the fact that my eyes were still closed and I was completely paralyzed. I have never been so terrified in my life. I KNEW someone else was in the room. I could hear them moving around. I felt like I was in grave danger. Then I KNOW I felt someone sit down on the bed right next to me! I tried to scream. . . . I was struggling and struggling but I couldn't even move a

8

finger. Finally, the episode passed and I woke up perfectly fine. I thought I was going crazy and never mentioned it to anyone. I still don't bring it up much because I get THAT LOOK from people who don't know what you're talking about. I have had several episodes since then. . . . I have never opened my eyes . . . and that is a blessing because if I ever did and saw something looking back at me I would probably die in my sleep. (Internet posting, Awareness during Sleep Paralysis Listserv [ASP-L])[2]

The Consistent Features of the Night-mare

The underlying structure of night-mares is strikingly similar around the globe, even in societies with no commonly accepted beliefs or traditions to offer cultural models for the experience. This similarity of night-mare accounts in vastly different contexts suggests that there is a uniform, core experience: the classic elements of the night-mare encounter are present regardless of cultural setting. I will describe these key characteristics individually, but they typically occur in clusters: (1) a sense of an evil presence accompanied by various sounds (footsteps, whispering); (2) breathing difficulties, feelings of suffocation, bodily pressure, sense of doom; and (3) sensations of floating, flying, and falling (including out-of-body experiences and viewing one's body from an external perspective). The first two clusters, which often co-occur, are characterized by intense terror and the third, although sometimes associated with fear, tends to be correlated with feelings of bliss (Cheyne 2005).

Being "Awake"

In recounting a night-mare experience, individuals go out of their way to emphasize that they were not sleeping during the attack: "I have suffered from sleep paralysis and it was the most scary thing in my life. The first time it happened I thought it was a dream but I know I was awake" (Internet posting, www.videojug.com). The terror of the event is heightened because it cannot be explained away as merely a frightening dream—it is experienced as a part of waking consciousness. Even after repeated episodes, the conviction of wakefulness cannot be shaken: "Each time is terrifying. I suddenly am awake and aware of the bed and my situation, but realize I cannot move. It is not a dream" (Internet posting, www.lakesidepress.com); "I am 'awake' during these attacks and even though at some point I can remind myself that it is [sleep paralysis], I CAN NOT talk myself down from the terror and panic I feel" (Internet posting, ASP-L).

Realistic Perception of Environment

Whether or not the victim remembers having his or her eyes open during a night-mare, the immediate environment is often realistically perceived: "I was aware of what was in the room . . . my memory is that I was awake and not asleep, not dreaming this with my eyes closed" (Adler, unpublished transcript); "I can sometimes see when having an episode. I can observe my dog sleeping on the floor. My husband lying beside me. My bedroom in general" (Internet posting, ASP-L). Perceiving "normal" surroundings realistically seems to add to the terror of the night-mare by confirming a waking state, and thus ruling out the possibility that the victim is merely dreaming and that the events are not "real."

Inability to Move

The sense of paralysis is often one of the first night-mare features noted in an episode: "I would wake up and I couldn't move and I couldn't breathe and there would be this terrifying struggle where I'd be trying to pull my arm up to my mouth to open my mouth, 'cause I'd think at the time that if I could just get my mouth open, I could breathe and I'd think that I would die if I could not do this" (Adler, unpublished transcript). The inability to move is sometimes attributed to an outside force: "I woke up, but I couldn't move for a while. I remember seeing my friend and his girlfriend and trying to say to them, 'I can't get up, someone is holding me down.' This was scary; I tried so hard to get up" (Internet posting, ASP-L); "I could feel something gripping me tighter and tighter and the more I resisted the tighter it became. I forced myself to try to move and, while being gripped, I could open my eyes and see, but could not move a muscle" (Internet posting, ASP-L).[3]

Overwhelming Fear and Dread

Another disturbing feature of the night-mare is the "overwhelming sense of dread/evil closing in." One victim describes having awakened many times in past years with a sense of "black horror": "[I] don't know any other way to describe it. I hate waking up at night, always afraid the figure will be back." In recounting the experience, people often have difficulty articulating the intensity of the horror they felt ("The fear progressed from foreboding to absolute panic") and may resort to descriptions of composite emotions ("Feelings of dread/bad/evil"). The emotion is "beyond" fear or terror, "like the evil is trying to reach my soul" (Internet postings, ASP-L).

Sensed Presence

The victim's feelings of horror/dread can be compounded by the awareness of an evil "presence," the sense that there is a watchful and malicious entity close by: "I just knew this presence was there. An ominous presence. And I was paralyzed—not only couldn't I—could I not see it, but I couldn't defend myself, I couldn't do anything, because I was paralyzed" (Adler, unpublished transcript).[4] When the sense of fear and the awareness of an entity co-occur, it is unclear whether the emotions of fear precede or result from the awareness of an evil presence, or whether they are inseparable.

> Many years back, I gathered some info on [sleep paralysis] . . . to show my father, who also suffers from [sleep paralysis]. (By the way, he is not an open minded person, whatsoever!) I had just learned of his experiences, and I wasn't aware that anyone else in my family had [sleep paralysis]. While sharing my new-found discoveries, my older brother (who far outweighs my father in disbelieving) relayed how as a child "he imagined" a "dark evil shadow" who would move throughout his room causing him great fear; so much so, that he was frozen and unable to move. I had never discussed this with my family prior to that day, or any other day thereafter. Sometimes, some subjects are best left alone and this was one of them. My point: there is something to this "dark presence." (Internet posting, ASP-L)

Chest Pressure

Just as paralysis can either be experienced discretely or understood as the result of restraint, chest pressure can be experienced as a decontextualized physical sensation of weight or understood to be caused by an entity crushing or pressing on the victim's chest. A typical account of the agent-free experience is a straightforward description of sensations: "I would wake up and feel this amazing pressure on my chest . . . and it was the sort—it was the sort of thing where it was so—it was so strong that I couldn't breathe" (Adler, unpublished transcript). When there is a crushing entity present, it may appear as a witch or other malevolent being (see illustration 1.1), but it may also manifest as a pressing force: "something invisible was trying to suffocate me" (Internet posting, ASP-L).

Difficulty Breathing

The sense of pressure on the chest is typically accompanied by difficulty breathing, although labored respiration can also occur without chest pressure.

> I was in the front passenger seat of my friend's truck, and we were wrapping up an 8 hour drive . . . the culmination of a 3-day ski weekend during which I skied hard, and slept little. So of course I was dozing on and off the whole way back. We stopped at our work, because he needed to run in and do some quick maintenance. So I stayed out in the truck to doze a bit. Judging by how I felt the last couple of short nods, I knew an episode was coming on, but I couldn't stop falling asleep. So it happened . . . and I could not move anything, breathing was either impossible or came in very short gasps that I could hear, and . . . I was aware of my surroundings, and was trying to claw my way out like I usually do. . . . The non-breathing is always the greatest fear, and the only reason I won't explore just letting

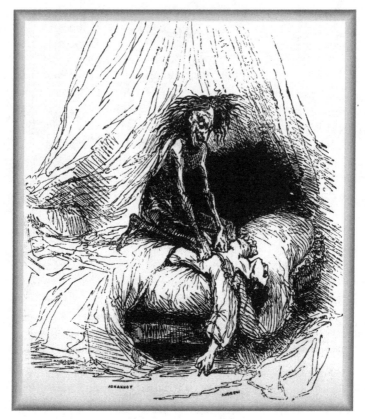

1.1. "Cauchemar," c. 1830. Engraving after Tony Johannot. Oxford, F. Haskell collection.

these happen. Eventually after 10 seconds or so, I clawed my way out and moved. I felt exhausted and out of breath. (Internet posting, ASP-L)

Supine Position

The majority of night-mares occur when the victim is sleeping on his or her back: "Mine happens when I'm in a supine position. After the event is over I'll usually turn and sleep on my side" (Internet posting, ASP-L). Although some sleep studies have shown that most people do not fall asleep on their backs, the majority of night-mares are experienced in that position (Cheyne 2002).

> I was asleep, on my back—I hardly ever sleep on my back—when it felt like something really heavy was on my chest and these really big hands were choking me. I couldn't breathe so I started struggling with it. My spouse reached over and began gently shaking me, asking if I was all right. When I opened my eyes this thing was ripping his hands off me. He looked like a gray, short, squatty gargoyle. I looked at my husband and back down

next to our bed and he was gone. This is the 1st time I have seen what was my attacker. And I was afraid to go back to sleep. When I did sleep it was in heavy short intervals. (Internet posting, ASP-L)

Additional Unusual Sensations

The victim of a night-mare may become aware of a range of unusual auditory, olfactory, or physical sensations. Examples of sounds include a door opening or closing, bedsprings creaking, an animal growling, approaching footsteps, rustling, or scratching. There may also be buzzing or beeping noises: "[My experience was] accompanied by a vibration or electric sound in my head that is like a humming or static (not sure if it is a noise or a feeling, maybe both?)" The individual may distinctly hear his or her name being called or may only be able to discern unintelligible—but clearly malevolent—whispering. Strange smells may also be a part of the experience, although they are much less common: "It smelled of death and decay or sorta like when a rat is dead in the attic or when cardboard gets wet and remains in a closed area"; "I could feel a cold, cold feeling running through me and a wicked smell, stench in the room." Finally, the "sleeper" may experience different types of motion, from the bed being lifted or covers being pulled off to bodily sensations of drifting, falling, or rolling: "[I] sometimes feel like I'm lying down on a roller coaster"; "I went flying down a tunnel really fast and wound up in a room just floating around it"; "I would feel my body rising up above my bed, and I would float there" (Internet postings, ASP-L).

The Night-mare in Language

The identifying features of the night-mare are evident in the terms used to refer to it. The etymology of the English word *nightmare,* for example, reveals a great deal about the experience itself. "Mare" comes from the same root as the German *mahr* and Old Norse *mara,* a supernatural being—usually female—who lay on people's chests at night, suffocating them (Kiessling 1968). The specific terms for night-mare that are used in many contemporary cultures are etymologically related to words for "weight" and "pressing." *Mare* appears to be of Indo-European origin, although its initial meaning is not clear. Linguists propose three possible roots of the word: *móros* ("death"), *mer* ("drive out"), and, perhaps the most likely source, *mar* ("to pound, bruise, crush") (Simpson and Weiner 1989). Because the sense of pressure or weight is prominent in the night-mare experience, it is not surprising that it is also a key element in the historical development of its linguistic forms. The idea of pressure is also present in other terms for the night-mare experience that do not share the *mare* linguistic root (see table 1.1). The medieval French *appesart* and the Spanish *pesadilla,* for example, are both derived from the verb *peser,* meaning "to press down upon" (Lecouteux 1987, cited in Davies 1996).

TABLE 1.1

Examples of Local, Cultural Terms for the Night-mare

Country	Local Term
Aceh (Indonesia) (Grayman, Good, and Good 2009)	*digeunton* ("pressed on"); *dicekek* ("choked or strangled)"
Arctic regions of Alaska, Canada, Greenland (Inuit) (Law and Kirmayer 2005)	*uqumangirniq; aqtuqsinniq*
Botswana (Mdlalani 2009)	*sebeteledi* ("someone who exerts pressure or force"); *setshitshama* ("that which paralyzes")
Cambodia (Hinton et al. 2005; Hinton et al. 2009)	*khmaoch sângkât* ("the ghost pushes you down")
China (Emmons 1982; Kingston 1989; Wing, Lee, and Chen 1994; Wing et al. 1999)	*bei guai chaak* ("being pressed by a ghost"); *bei gui ya* ("held by a ghost")
Czech Republic (Boiadjiev and Müller 2003)	*muera*
Egypt (Mandhur 2006; Sayce 1900)	*al-Jathoom* (<yajthum, "sits"); *kabus* (<incubus)
Estonia (Davies 2003)	*luupainaja* ("the one who presses your bones")
Finland (Davies 2003)	*painajainen* (<painaa, "to press or apply pressure")
France (Rickels 1961; Roberts 1998)	*cauchemar* (<caucher, "to tread on")
Germany (Boiadjiev and Müller 2003; Ward 1977, 1981)	*Alpdruck* ("elf pressure"); *Hexendrucken* ("witch pressing"); *Nachtmahr*
Hungary (Davies 2003; Schonberger 1946)	*boszorkany-nyomas* ("witches' pressure"); *lidércnyomás* (nyomás = "pressing")
Iceland (Davies 2003)	*martröd* (<troda, "to squeeze, press, ride")
Ireland (Dolan 2006)	*tromluí; tromlaige* ("being pressed upon")

(Continued)

TABLE 1.1

(Continued)

Country	Local Term
Italy (Boiadjiev and Müller 2003)	*pesuarole* (<*pesante* = "weight"); *incubo*
Japan (Arikawa et al. 1999; Fukuda et al. 1998; Schegoleva 2002)	*kanashibari* ("bound or fastened by metal")
Korea (Firestone 1985)	*ka-wi-nulita* ("scissors pressed")
Laos (Lao PDR) (Heimbach 1979), United States (Adler 1991, 1994; Bliatout 2003)	*dab tsog, tsog tsuam* ("to crush, press, or smother")
Mexico (Foster 1973; Jacobson 2009; Jiménez-Genchi et al. 2009)	*pesadilla*
Morocco (de Jong 2005)	*boratat* ("someone who presses on you")
Netherlands (Bremmer, Johnston, and Vries 1998; Davies 2003)	*nachtmerrie*
Newfoundland (Hufford 1982; Ness 1978)	*Old Hag, ag rog* ("hag ridden")
Norway (Davies 2003)	*mareritt*
Poland (Boiadjiev and Müller 2003; Kiessling 1968)	*zmora*
Portugal (de Jong 2005)	*pesadelo* (<pesado, "heavy")
Republic of Croatia (Davies 2003)	*morica*
Russia (Hufford 1982; Montagu-Nathan 1917)	*kikimora*
Thailand (Firestone 1985)	*phi um* ("ghost covered"); *phi kau* ("ghost possessed")

(Continued)

TABLE 1.1

(Continued)

Country	Local Term
Turkey (Rønnevig 2007)	*karabasan* ("dark presser")
West Indies (Ness 1978)	*kokma*
Zanzibar (Walsh 2009)	*popobawa* ("bat wing"—from dark shadow cast by the spirit when it attacks)

Three Examples of the Night-mare in Contemporary Cultural Settings

The core night-mare phenomenon is stable across cultures, although, as a consequence of variations in experience and context, its significance and impact vary considerably: despite the remarkable stability of the night-mare syndrome and its universal distribution, culture-specific elaborations do exist. In most instances, cultural factors appear to shape the encounter, as well as the experience and interpretation of it (Hufford 1982). There are myriad examples of contemporary night-mare traditions. I will present three brief "case studies"—Newfoundlander, Inuit, and Japanese—in order to illustrate the night-mare's widespread geographical and cultural distribution.

The Old Hag of Newfoundland

In the early 1970s, David J. Hufford became a faculty member of the Folklore Department at Memorial University of Newfoundland. At that time, Newfoundland had a small population for whom "the conservative influences of isolation . . . left intact . . . elements of traditional culture no longer functioning in most of the English-speaking world" (Hufford 1982, 1). Hufford was primarily interested in folk belief and was able, through his archival duties and subsequent fieldwork, to study accounts of ghosts, fairies, and omens of death. He first encountered the Newfoundland night-mare, "the Old Hag," while investigating these traditions. Hufford eventually collected hundreds of examples of Old Hag attacks, all of which share the same basic features. As one twenty-year-old university student described the phenomenon: "You are dreaming and you feel as if someone is holding you down. You can do nothing, only cry out. People believe that you will die if you're not awakened" (Hufford 1982, 2).

Through a survey conducted at Memorial University in 1971, Hufford found that about 15 percent of students were familiar with the tradition that described the Old Hag. The experience was considered to include the features of awakening, hearing and/or seeing something come into the room and approach the bed, being pressed on the chest or strangled, and being unable to move or cry out (1982, 10–11). Newfoundlanders referred to the victim of an Old Hag attack as having been "hag rid," that is, ridden by the Hag (which causes the pressure or crushing sensation on the chest). Hufford draws an intriguing connection between the pronunciation of "hag rid" and "haggard" and explains that the Newfoundland usage may represent one step in the etymology of the word, since *haggard* is now used generally to refer to someone who appears worried and fatigued (Hufford 1982, 54–55)—precisely the way one would expect someone who had been ridden by the Old Hag to look.

In addition to the systematic documentation of the Old Hag as a common and living tradition in Newfoundland, perhaps Hufford's greatest contribution to the study of the night-mare is his explanation of the experience's potential source.

> I immediately knew that "the Old Hag" broke the conventional rules about cultural shaping. In 1967, before ever visiting Newfoundland, I had heard the footsteps, sensed the terrifying presence and felt it climb onto *my* chest, all the while unable to move or cry out. I didn't talk with any-one about it. . . . I had no idea that it had ever happened to anyone else. Now I found that Newfoundlanders knew all about "my experience." Sleep paralysis incorporating a threatening spiritual presence could not reflect simple cultural loading, because I lacked the cultural background to produce the "traditional" details that I had experienced. My experi-ence in 1967 had felt "spiritual," although I had not believed in malevo-lent spirits. . . . Meeting the Old Hag in Newfoundland several years after my own encounter felt like independent confirmation of my unwilling "observations." (Hufford 2005, 19)

At the time of Hufford's Newfoundland research, sleep paralysis and hypnagogic hallucinations were both little studied and poorly understood sleep disorders (Chambers 1999). In the quarter century since the publication of Hufford's sem-inal work, *The Terror That Comes in the Night,* much more has been learned about these parasomnias, and many people—myself included—are convinced that Hufford is correct in identifying Old Hag attacks with them. Hufford's research in Newfoundland laid the foundation for thinking of the night-mare as truly universal and experience-centered, rather than merely the result of a culture-based phenomenon that arises independently in different parts of the world.

The Uqumangirniq *of Canada*

> Just before I fall asleep I get paralyzed. Sometimes it starts with a hum-
> ming sound. Sometimes I can hardly see and I get scared. My grandpar-
> ents told me it was a ghost trying to get hold of me and they said I should
> fight against it. After the humming sound I cannot move anymore.
> Sometimes it feels as if I am not inside but outside my body, as if I have
> to fight to get back in. When I do not return immediately I do not man-
> age to go back any more and it feels like I could die. At those times, I
> really panic. Sometimes it feels like an eternity before I can move again. I
> finally wake up with a pounding heart and I feel all shaken up and I'm
> frightened. (Bloom and Gelardin 1976, 21)

The Inuit of Canada have a rich set of concepts and vocabulary to describe
night-mare phenomena, and the terms for the experience vary across the
region. In the Baffin dialect, the night-mare is called *uqumangirniq;* in the
Kivalliq region, the term is *aqtuqsinniq:* "When you are sleeping and you are
unable to move. You can't stand up. You can't move. That's what we mean by
aqtuqsinniq. It is the same thing as *uqumangirniq.* They say that some people do
not wake up from *aqtuqsinniq*" (Kolb and Law 2001, 190).

In the late 1990s, the Inuit-led Nunavut Arctic College sponsored a project
designed to preserve traditional Inuit cultural knowledge. As part of this
endeavor, anthropologist Stephane Kolb and psychiatrist Samuel Law interviewed Inuit elders, adults, and young people in order to record and study their
collective oral history. Dreams and their interpretations were a prominent
theme in the interviews and a source of fascination for many of the college's
faculty and students. Kolb and Law learned that there is a widespread belief
that *siniktuq* ("sleep") is a state in which people make contact with the invisible spirit world, the world of the dead. *Uqumangirniq* is part of this shamanistic
cosmology.

In Inuit tradition, people are comprised of three souls: the *tarniq,* which is
indestructible (and sometimes described as a bubble that floats within the body
but can exist free of the body); the breath soul, which animates the body and
disappears at death; and the name soul, which is carried in the name and
bestowed on someone through the act of naming. The *tarniq* of the living, especially children, is considered delicate: Inuit elders believe that when the *tarniq*
is in a vulnerable state, *uqumangirniq* can result from an attack by a shaman or
malevolent spirit. In sleep and dreams, the relationship between an individual
and his or her *tarniq* becomes weak and fragile. Sickness can result from a person's *tarniq* straying too far from his or her physical body: "If a person's *tarniq*
were to leave the body while the person was sleeping, the *tarniq* would be able
to see the body it had just left behind. The body would appear hollow, as if it had
no insides. . . . If the *tarniq* had really left the body behind the person would die.

Our body is just a casing for our *tarniq*" (Kolb and Law 2001, 35). As an Inuit elder describes:

> There was one time I was in bed with my wife and I couldn't wake up at all. There was an old man wearing caribou clothing. . . . This old man was standing between us and was smiling at me and reaching towards me. His face was healthy and handsome but it started to become older. He became ugly and he seemed to have lots of hair. Because I remembered what my grandmother had told me to do, I stuck my finger up at him. I seemed to feel him, and then he fell backwards and disappeared. I thought this had come from someone and I didn't want to die. I started wondering, "Why are Tautunngi and Qabluittug's [acquaintances] son doing this to me?" Then I thought, "I have hit his *tarniq*. Maybe he won't live." (Kolb and Law 2001, 189)

Uqumangirniq is a state of awareness experienced when one awakens, but is paralyzed. People commonly hear hissing, roaring, or humming sounds preceding or during this paralysis: "To me, it is never going to stop being scary. I think when you experience this you are scared every time. It is scarier when your ears hiss, as this means there is something very close to you. When I was still a child, I thought I was going to die. I really wanted to move my body but I couldn't" (Kolb and Law 2001, 192). Unusual visual perceptions during *uqumangirniq* are also reported, sometimes with a sense of someone approaching: "He was wearing a very thin sinew belt. He was not wearing his *kamiik* [sealskin boots]. He was wearing mitts made out of caribou foreleg. I thought maybe he had been sent to me. I was lying in bed and his face became uglier and uglier and he seemed to get closer and closer" (Kolb and Law 2001, 192).

Despite the range of details, the terror associated with *uqumangirniq* is unmistakable; the greatest fear is that one will never awaken again. Although Kolb and Law did not attempt to determine the incidence of *uqumangirniq*, it appeared to be well-known and easily recognized. Inuit elders, however, expressed concern that this knowledge was being lost and the information threatened by the profound shift in Inuit beliefs during their lifetime. The elders lamented the passing of the time when shamans were able to help and protect their communities.

In contrast to Inuit elders' understandings of *uqumangirniq* from within a traditional Inuit religious context, younger Inuit invoked Christian beliefs, particularly the notion of the "devil." One woman related: "When I was 14, I had my first *uqumangirniq*. . . . The devil tried to get to me. It had no face, no shape. Evil. I couldn't move, couldn't run, like I was in a weakened state. I prayed: 'Leave me, in the name of Jesus.' It really worked. My words came out slowly" (Kolb and Law 2001, 208–209). Although some *uqumangirniq* accounts contained mixed references to both Christian "devils" and shamanistic entities, there was a nearly

complete shift from the elders' shamanistic cosmology to the younger generations' Christian references to satanic entities.

This new trend in understanding and interpretation is not surprising,
given the profound influence Christianity has had in Arctic Canada in the last
century (Dorais 1997; Fletcher and Kirmayer 1997). Kolb and Law note that, in
the early 1990s, members of Inuit communities were reluctant to talk about
shamanism because it was associated with pre-Christian traditions they had
come to disavow as part of their Christian identities. Some missionaries
explained that traditional Inuit beliefs were not so much untrue as they were
evidence of the workings of the devil. "Beneath this discourse on demonic
possession and the actions of the devil it is possible to discern traces of older
shamanistic tradition but this was not actively endorsed as such by most Inuit
interviewed" (Fletcher and Kirmayer 1997, 202). It is only in the last decade
that there has been "renewed interest and pride among younger Inuit in
recovering traditional knowledge including shamanic tradition" (Law and
Kirmayer 2005, 109). Traditional knowledge still plays a role in contemporary
interpretations, but, for younger Inuit, traditional interpretations have been
almost entirely supplanted by Christian, secular, and scientific accounts.
Despite the fact that shamanism is no longer practiced widely, it still serves as
a powerful explanatory model for some segments of Inuit society (Kolb and
Law 2001).

The Kanashibari *of Japan*

The night-mare is a well-known phenomenon in Japan; it has been experienced
by at least one-third of the population, and most people are familiar with the
Japanese term for the encounter, *kanashibari* (Arikawa et al. 1999; Fukuda et al.
1998). During an attack, victims of *kanashibari* cannot move and often see an
intruder entering their room and sitting or lying on top of them; the experience
is typically accompanied by intense fear or anxiety (see illustration 1.2).
Kanashibari literally means "bound (or fastened) in metal" (*kana* = "metal";
shibaru = "to bind, tie, fasten") and refers to the victim's paralysis. In 2001,
researcher Anna Schegoleva interviewed ten- to twelve-year-old Japanese schoolchildren about the night-mare phenomenon. The children she interviewed
knew the term *kanashibari* from computer games, television programs, books,
friends, and (much less frequently) family members.

> It happened when I was five. I remember lying in my bed, my body being
> pressed by someone in long white clothes. I could see my brother sleep-
> ing but could not move to free myself or scream for help.
>   Was it a male or female figure?
> I immediately decided that it was a female. I don't know why.
>   You remember it quite well. How did it end?

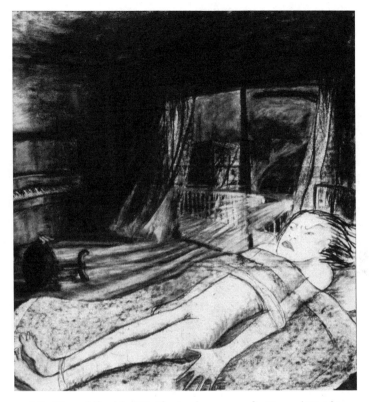

1.2. "Kanashibari," 1986. Charcoal on paper, by Kazumi Honda.

I felt that I could move my toes, and the same moment the ghost disappeared.

Do you think it was a ghost?

My brother told me next morning: so you had *kanashibari* and saw a ghost! (Schegoleva 2002, 31)

Schegoleva found that the physical experiences of the children were consistent: pressure on the chest (or all over the body), immobility, and breathing difficulties. Variations are restricted to sounds and visual manifestations. The most common night-mare intruders include: Sadako (from the *Ringu* book and movie—a female figure in white clothes, limping up to the sleeper, with long, dark hair concealing her face), ghosts, and unfamiliar people. Some children see the same figure every time, but others see different people (for example, "strangers" who come through their bedroom windows and then stare at them as they lie in bed, paralyzed with fear).

Unlike other industrialized societies, including the United States, the medical term "sleep paralysis" is well known in Japan. Even so, night-mare entities are widely believed to be the spirits of the dead, the most feared of which is the *kanashibari*. As a Japanese college student describes:

> In the middle of the night, I suddenly found out that something or some-one was upon me, on my bed. Every time I tried to get up, he pushed me down. And I couldn't move an inch and I couldn't cry for help, because, somehow, my voice didn't come. I felt that the thing tried to absorb my strength. I even felt the face of the thing just in front of me. And, still, I was completely awake. So I don't think any scientific explanation explains that kind of experience, that fear. (Gray and Gray 2008)

Schoolchildren report different causes for *kanashibari*. It can be nighttime punishment for behaving unkindly toward others during the day, but it can also be caused by studying too much at night so that one's usual sleep patterns are disrupted. Attacks can happen during daytime naps as well. In contrast to Newfoundlander and Inuit night-mare traditions, experiencing *kanashibari* and subsequently sharing the terrifying details of the encounter are seen as desirable by many Japanese children (and college students). Some devise strategies and techniques for luring *kanashibari*. Children generally understand that sleeping in a supine position is a prerequisite for the attacks. They believe that falling asleep while clutching a favorite toy or going to bed crying are also likely to cause *kanashibari*. When Schegoleva inquired into means for avoiding *kanashibari*, her young interviewees were too eager to experience the night-mare to devise means for staying away from it. (Some Japanese college students' Web logs include descriptions of their *kanashibari* experiences as a part of their everyday lives. Visitors describe how much they enjoy the horror of the experience.)

In Japan, both children and adults experience *kanashibari* in the context of a strong mass media influence. The night-mare experience is so widely recog-nized that it is the subject of television programs and *manga* (Japanese graphic novels). In one television program about *kanashibari*, celebrity Kitano Takeshi was comically tied to a chair with metal chains while he cried for help; similar representations are sometimes used in both television dramas and comedies (Schegoleva 2002; Terrillon and Marques-Bonham 2001).

Preventing and Escaping Night-mare Attacks

Across cultures, night-mare attacks are variously attributed to supernatural causes (e.g., evil spirits, spirits of the dead, envious or malicious living people, supernatural animals); natural causes (overindulging in food or drink before bed, indigestion, fatigue, stress, poor circulation, sleeping on one's back);[5] or any combination of these factors. In all three sample cases of contemporary night-mare manifestations—Newfoundlander, Inuit, and Japanese—as well as in many other cultural settings, naturalistic and supernatural explanations for night-mare causes coexist.

Where there is a shared tradition of the night-mare assault, there are not only widely known explanations regarding its cause, but also means of preventing or escaping its clutches. These strategies are not always successful, but, at a minimum, they serve to contextualize and give meaning to the experience. Making an effort not to sleep on one's back is perhaps the most universal of the prophylactic measures. In Sweden, there is also a custom of not peering through a keyhole or knot-hole before retiring to bed, since the night-mare spirit usually enters through these types of openings. For the same reason, closing every possible opening to the bedroom is desirable (Tillhagen 1969, 318, 326). There is an Afro-Caribbean practice of putting a broom in the bedroom at night, because the night-mare witch (*kokma*) will be compelled to count the straws and thus unable to "ride" the sleeper (Paradis and Friedman 2005). In order to prevent *uqumangirniq,* Inuit elders emphasize the importance of avoiding conflicts—especially with shamans—confessing wrongdoing, and being respectful and kind to others. In addition, it is important to talk to children about *uqumangirniq* in order to transmit knowledge of its meaning and the methods of self-protection. Some younger Inuit advocate additional forms of prevention, including telling others about *uqumangirniq* attacks as soon as possible, changing sleep positions, praying, putting a Bible under the pillow, putting an *ulu* (knife) under the pillow, going to confession and receiving blessings at church, and talking to elders.

In the event that avoidance maneuvers are unsuccessful (or could not be attempted), there are several strategies for escaping the night-mare. One apparently universal belief is that, by making the smallest motion with a finger or toe, the victim can put an end to the attack. Accomplishing even the slightest movement drives the night-mare away and allows the "sleeper" to recover immediately. Among people who consider a night-mare to be a bewitched person, there is the belief that it is possible to escape by rattling names off quickly; when the correct name is mentioned, the night-mare is forced to adopt human form (Tillhagen 1969). When the night-mare is caused by a malicious human being, identifying the true identity of the spirit will destroy its power. There are also specific charms that, if spoken to a night-mare spirit during an attack, will end the ordeal: "If one can say to the Night-mare, '*Trud,* come in the morrow/for something to borrow,' then the spirit will have to flee, but it will return in the morning in the shape of a human in order to borrow something" (Ward 1981, I, 91). As a last resort, there are traditional instructions to be carried out when a person becomes aware of a night-mare attack on someone nearby. With the Inuit, a person who witnesses another experiencing *uqumangirniq* is expected to help. In Newfoundland, people who have observed Old Hag attacks report that "touching or shaking the victim would bring them out of it" (Ness 1978).

The Night-mare Outside of a Shared Tradition

The basic features of the night-mare are remarkably consistent around the world, although various groups interpret and describe their similar experiences in different ways. Researchers have come to believe that because the fundamental experience of the night-mare is consistent across time and locale, cultural accounts of the night-mare are grounded in actual events. In other words, the night-mare encounter may be culturally elaborated upon before, during, and after the experience, but culture is not the source of the event. If cultural models provided all of the content for night-mare encounters, members of a sociocultural group might be expected to share similar experiences, but it does not follow that people with different (or no) cultural traditions of the night-mare would encounter the same phenomenon randomly.

In spite of the clear universality of the night-mare, before Hufford and others began to focus on its experiential core, researchers looking at individual or local instances of attacks assumed that they were culture-specific; night-mares were considered to be a recognizable "syndrome" only within a specific society or culture. The American Psychiatric Association characterizes this type of disorder as a "culture-bound syndrome" (a concept that remains highly controversial): "Generally limited to specific societies or culture areas," these "are localized, folk, diagnostic categories that have coherent meanings for certain repetitive, patterned, and troubling sets of experiences and observations" (1994, 844). Although the night-mare manifests locally, neither the distribution nor the subjective content of night-mare attacks depend on cultural knowledge of the phenomenon. The basic features of accounts given by men and women from Newfoundland, for example, are indistinguishable from Inuit or Japanese retellings. Only the specifics of interpretation (such as the nature and the cultural details of the entity) vary substantially. Night-mares also appear with similar frequency in different settings, although they are reported much less freely in the absence of cultural explanatory frameworks. For these reasons, the night-mare does not comprise a culture-bound syndrome.

Although culture is not the source of the experience, cultural beliefs do play an important role in determining the degree of salience of the night-mare. In the absence of an explanatory framework, many night-mare sufferers have no idea that others report such encounters and are, understandably, hesitant to share their own experiences. Yet, despite the fact that these individuals have no ancient or widely shared tradition to draw on, their accounts can be readily identified by anyone familiar with one of those traditions (see illustration 1.3). This is precisely what has occurred in my own experience. I had four or five episodes of sleep paralysis in my early twenties—all limited to a sense of paralysis, difficulty breathing, and a sort of "creepy" feeling. I had no cultural framework

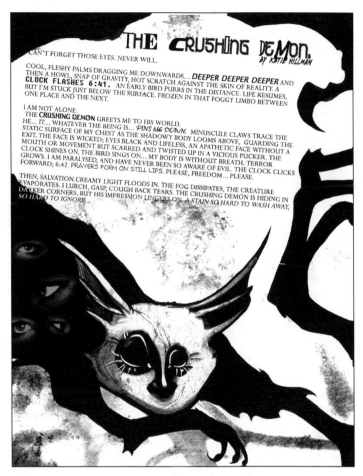

1.3. "The Crushing Demon," 2008. Digital art, by Katie Hillman.

for the experience, including no readily available explanation for the event, and subsequently interpreted the night-mare as an extremely unpleasant but "natural" occurrence.

In the summer of 1987, I was staying with my aunt in Jerusalem, preparing to begin fieldwork on local night-mare experiences. Late one night, I was startled awake, not by a night-mare, but by a human intruder—a police officer who had mistaken my sleeping form for that of an elusive suspect he was in the process of tracking from house to house. For obvious reasons, I had difficulty falling back asleep after his departure. I soon found myself unable to move or breathe, and this one time I sensed an entity: a clearly evil presence that, after a few moments, transformed visually into a figure (bearing an uncanny resemblance to *Mad* magazine's Alfred E. Neuman). Both the "entity" and paralysis disappeared after a few seconds, but—despite my immersion in sleep paralysis research—they left a strong and disturbing impression.

The project I was conducting in Israel in the late 1980s was an interview study with recent immigrants on the topic of sleep experiences. Out of forty people with whom I spoke, seven had experienced at least one night-mare, yet none of the participants was familiar with any cultural traditions regarding the experience. My exploratory study focused on representations of the night-mare in this absence of explicit cultural models. The seven participants characterized their experiences in a variety of ways: one man explained that the event felt like breathing exercises (to warm up before singing) that had gone awry, leaving him helpless and gasping for air; one woman felt that her cat had climbed up on her chest while she was sleeping and prevented normal respiration; another man believed that there was a potential murderer in the room; and four people (one man and three women) who were living near Gaza at the time of the beginning of the first Intifada (1987), visualized the night-mare as a Palestinian intruder. From conversations with Palestinian men and women who described the night-mares of relatives living in refugee camps, it was clear that—in the visualization of night-mare intruders—the reverse was also true: some Palestinians, especially adolescent boys, visualized night-mare attacks as intrusions by Israeli soldiers. Under certain conditions, it seems, the mind of an individual trapped in this terrifying waking/sleeping state struggles to make sense of the dilemma by postulating an attacker consistent with readily available alternatives.

Cultural elaboration, although driven by the phenomenology of sleep paralysis, clearly follows preexisting models. Thus, in Japan, *kanashibari* provides evidence of the presence of the spirit world. In the United States, however, the night-mare is often experienced apart from a shared cultural tradition and outside of a readily identifiable explanatory framework. Since the strange and compelling nature of sleep paralysis demands explanation, the experience "may encourage interpretations in terms of the extraordinary or uncanny and lend conviction to accounts that would otherwise seem far-fetched" (Hinton, Hufford, and Kirmayer 2005, 9). People who experience the night-mare in environments that do not provide traditional cultural explanations rely on a variety of alternative strategies to make sense of the encounter. In order to learn how people understand their night-mares in the contemporary United States, I have closely followed Internet postings and discussions for the past several years. It is clear that people who have night-mares outside of a cultural framework of understanding draw upon a contemporary narrative in interpreting their experiences—such as one derived from medicine or psychiatry (for example, heart disease or mental illness), religion (demons), or the paranormal (including alien abductions)—or they construct their own personal narrative. Perhaps equally intriguing is the fact that many people who experience sleep paralysis find that the condition holds no great significance for them.[6]

Fears of Physical or Mental Illness

In societies in which the night-mare is not widely acknowledged or discussed, its dramatic symptoms are sometimes mistaken for evidence of physical or mental illness. The absence of shared personal accounts of these experiences can be misleading, giving the impression that they do not occur in the mainstream, "normal" American population. Forty years ago, for example, a physician reported that "people, especially after they have had several attacks, are afraid it's a premonitory sign of some dreadful brain disease, maybe a tumor or a stroke. One man came to me with the complaint, 'I have seizures in my sleep.' He had classical attacks of postdormital paralysis and he thought it was epilepsy" (Levin 1967, 1229). Today, general ignorance of the symptoms of sleep paralysis is still evident among both night-mare sufferers and the medical community: "My doctor was of no help to me and she referred me to a neurologist and neither of them had ever heard of [sleep paralysis]. I had a CAT scan done and my brain was normal—I was afraid I had a brain tumor" (Internet posting, ASP-L). People's concerns are not limited to "physical disease," however; the most frequently reported fear is that the nocturnal experiences are symptoms of mental illness: "I feel like I am going crazy, plain and simple"; "[I'm] just wondering if any of these occurrences with the dark side have anything to do with mental illness. I see my meetings with the invisible, paralyzing man that tortures me as possible bipolar hallucinations" (Internet postings, ASP-L). These concerns are only intensified when physicians are unfamiliar with sleep paralysis symptoms. One night-mare sufferer urged patients to be prepared to educate their health care practitioners: "Go armed with info, as my doctor referred me to a psychiatrist" (Internet posting, ASP-L).

When personal accounts of night-mare attacks are not widely shared, enormous relief comes with the realization that others recognize one's experience. The easing of night-mare sufferers' distress upon hearing of others' accounts is so great that it forms a motif in almost all initial disclosures. It is very common to hear, "I thought I was the only person in the world that this happened to" (Adler, unpublished transcript). The discovery of shared experiences is especially powerful in contemporary American society because the lack of general acknowledgment of night-mares increases the impact of "corroborating" accounts. The following exchange, on a sleep paralysis listserv, exemplifies both the isolation felt by night-mare sufferers and their related fears of mental illness:

> [Initial posting] I have told my parents about all of them but they don't believe me and I have no idea what any of this means. I'm still confused about [sleep paralysis] and the whole paralysis thing. I just know I've seen some crazy things and I have no idea what they mean. I just now read about this and it seems pretty close to what I've seen but I dunno. They might just be made up in my head and that's what I'm trying to find out.

[*Reply*] I understand this one. I was probably a bit older than you when my [sleep paralysis] started (I was 23) and when I told my mum she freaked out and said I was being punished for some kind of wrongdoing in the past. I didn't find out until nearly 20 years later that my dad, my grandmother, and one of my uncles had it, too, but the family had been keeping it secret because they thought it was a sign of insanity!

I know it's hard when your parents don't believe you, but you have to try and see it from their point of view. If you'd heard about [sleep paralysis] before it started happening to you, you probably wouldn't have believed it either! You're going to have to be very adult about this and try to protect them for the time being, or they'll end up getting worried about you and that won't help anyone. There's at least 200 of us on this list, all of whom you can talk to, either in public or offlist. Read all the posts, ask as many questions as you like, and once you've got it straight in your own head, you'll find it easier to talk to your parents about it. And don't worry about those "crazy things" you're seeing. They're hallucinations, they can't hurt you, and it doesn't mean *you're* crazy. Almost everyone on this list sees, hears, or feels crazy things when they're paralysed and we're all still here and still sane! (Internet posting, ASP-L)

This discussion also illustrates the central role of experience, rather than culture, in the core features. Since the young man who began this thread did not realize, at the time of his first night-mare, that others have similar attacks, he was not culturally predisposed to believe in them.

Religious and Spiritual Interpretations

It must be more than the lack of common terminology or acknowledgment of shared experience that account for the fact that the night-mare is not more widely recognized in a society like that of the United States. Since other groups of people, with similar rates of sleep paralysis, continue to maintain an explanatory context for the night-mare, one possible explanation is that, while there is a "strong tendency for sleep paralysis to be experienced as a kind of spiritual experience," there is a "tension between spiritual experience and modern medicine, and modern views of spirituality and religion in general" (Hufford 2005, 12). The biomedical premise that direct spiritual experiences are psychopathological, as well as the mainstream religious view that they are heretical, suppresses the reporting and discussing of night-mare encounters. Louis Proud, an Australian writer and researcher of paranormal and occult phenomena, writes of his first sleep paralysis attack:

When I was seventeen years old something changed within my mind; a shift of awareness occurred, and I became receptive to the presence of invisible beings—and I still am. Call them spirits if you like. Whenever I hear, feel, see, and sense these beings, I am always in an altered state of consciousness. Never am I fully awake. I do not have, and have never had, any kind of mental illness, nor am I on medication for any reason whatsoever; nor do I take recreational drugs. (Proud 2009, 15)

The author's need to establish his experiences as unrelated to either a psychological disorder or psychoactive substance is evidence of the marginalization of "nonstandard" scientific or religious interpretations. Yet many, if not most, night-mare sufferers in the United States interpret their experiences as having at least a spiritual component. The following account of a demonic night-mare attack was posted on a Web site "where you can find all kinds of resources regarding real ghosts and true haunting cases, but more importantly, it is a site for publishing, sharing, and reading real ghost stories from real people like you."[7]

One Saturday morning, I woke up tired, cranky, irritable and just did not want to work. I did not feel like packing any boxes [to help my sister move] or cleaning or sweeping, I just didn't. . . . So as I'm laying there on the bed (it was about 10:30 am) I suddenly could not move. I could not scream and I could not think. One thing I could do was HEAR and I heard two distinct voices: one was a demonic woman that said "We should have never let you get away from us"—then a demonic man's voice that said "This time you will not get away from us." I struggled and struggled and felt my mouth moving and calling my sister—actually I know I was screaming her name—but she was downstairs in the garage and could in no way hear me. After what seemed like an eternity, the pressure suddenly left and I got up. I ran downstairs and asked [my sister] if she could hear me calling her name, she said No. I told her what happened and she said why didn't you pray to God? I said that I couldn't think, I was just too scared and it caught me off guard. To this day I wonder who the heck those demons were and what they meant by "we should have never let you get away from us." . . . [Now] I actually talk down the demons that are attacking me and act like some sort of super hero. I rebuke them in the name of Jesus Christ and it always works, they are defeated. For all of you who have been having this happen to you, I notice that none of you rebuke the demons but instead try to fight them off or scream. Rebuking them in the name of Jesus Christ will send them fleeing, trust me, they are powerful words. I've always felt that there is some kind of power struggle going on for my soul. . . . Remember the words "I rebuke you in the name of Jesus Christ." . . . Say it over and over and say it loudly even if you can only say it in your head . . . People, please put on your suit of armor and don't be demon doormats anymore. (Internet posting, www.yourghoststories.com)

This young woman's description of her encounters is part of a distinctly Christian subset of night-mare experiences. Although these encounters are experienced outside of a cultural tradition of night-mares, they do fit well within an evangelical Christian worldview. A young man similarly describes nocturnal attacks by demons:

> I'm glad to hear that others experience this. It started when I was in my mid teens. I had recently become a Christian when I woke up one night paralyzed with fear. I just know that there was a demon in my room even though I hadn't seen anything. When I started praying I noticed that the presence diminished. I quickly learned that whenever this happened, praying was the best weapon. A few years back this became very frequent, almost nightly. One time I even felt something jump on me, then jump off. It was not heavy. It reminded me of a cat jumping on me. At that point, I said "That's IT!" I got out of bed and prayed audibly, casting out the demons from my home and told them they were not welcome to come back. It was almost a comical sight. Guess what? It stopped that very night. Some people think this is medical. I'm not so sure! (Internet posting, www.websciences.org)

Interestingly, although these attacks have clear religious implications, the accounts—and many others like them—were not posted on religious Web sites; they were described on discussion boards devoted to ghost stories or sleep phenomena. Knowing that the event is considered by some to be sleep paralysis was interesting to these writers, but did not change their religious interpretation of the encounters. The tension between religious experience and biomedicine is recognized, but it is not sufficiently compelling—when compared to the actual experience of the night-mare—to challenge the perception that the experiences are demon driven. Similarly, the fact that sleep paralysis is becoming more widely known does not diminish the spiritual impact of night-mares for many people. As Louis Proud writes:

> I've thought long and hard about the importance of . . . the sleep paralysis phenomenon. . . . There exists another reality—a "spirit realm"— impinging upon our own, whose inhabitants influence us profoundly and play a much larger role in our lives than we care to imagine—or are able to comprehend. Being a sleep paralysis sufferer has enabled me to become aware of this reality, not in an abstract sense, but in a factual sense. It has also enabled me to realize that the soul exists and can be understood. . . . I realize, of course, that many of us—perhaps most of the world's population—believe in some kind of spirit realm or afterlife and also accept the existence of the soul. However, when I say that the sleep

paralysis phenomenon has enabled me to find my soul, I'm doing much more than simply acknowledging my spirituality, or implying that I've had a "spiritual awakening." You could have a "spiritual awakening" as a result of frolicking naked through a field of poppies on a spring morning. I'm using the word "soul" in a very literal sense. As I'm sure many sleep paralysis sufferers would agree, the sleep paralysis state puts you in direct contact with your soul, allowing you to experience the spirit realm first-hand. This is immensely significant—even revolutionary. (Proud 2009, 268)

For some people, the terror of the encounter can thus occasionally be ameliorated by what is considered to be an opportunity for spiritual growth.

Paranormal Interpretations

The term "alien abduction" refers to the kidnapping of human beings by extraterrestrial creatures and the temporary removal of the victims from their earthly surroundings. There is considerable variation among alien abduction accounts, but many fit a common pattern. The experience often begins at night, when the person is at home in bed (Spanos et al. 1993; Spanos et al. 1995; Wright 1994), though sometimes abductions occur from a car or outdoors. The abductee awakens from sleep with a feeling of dread or a sense of a presence in the room. The bedroom may be flooded with light that is often accompanied by a buzzing or humming sound. The aliens either come to get the abductee or the victim is transported or "floated" to a spacecraft. Once inside the craft, the person may be subjected to various medical procedures that typically involve the removal of eggs or sperm. (The aliens' purpose in abducting human beings varies in different accounts, but it often involves the creation of a breeding program—necessitating the extraction of human gametes in order to produce alien-human hybrids.) The human victim feels helpless and is often restrained or partially or completely paralyzed during the encounter (Blackmore 1998; Chambers 1999).

> Once I was conscious, and I saw a kind of "nurse" very near my face, like looking at something, or maybe inducing a kind of mental order. I was so mad cause I couldn't move. It was not a dream, even if it seems a dream. I was fighting a lot to move my arm, and with all my strength I could raise it. Then the "nurse" moved backwards, but I was so weak, it took a tremendous effort to just move my arm. I felt like a puppet, controlled by these beings. But not all aliens do this kind of thing, and it was not an [out-of-body experience], cause the "nurse" moved backwards when I raised my arm, as if astonished because I could move. (Internet posting, ASP-L)

Not all aliens are viewed as evil; sometimes the encounters are quite benign, with the entities, for example, warning against harm to the environment. Some people view these experiences as pleasant or even transformative.

> I've had a similar experience with 'Grays' [humanoid extraterrestrials]. I had them all around my bed. Interestingly enough, when I sat up they all jumped backwards in unison. That did not stop them on the other hand transporting through the wall of the apartment and up into a spacecraft that must have been, by my reckoning, about a mile in diameter. I remember I could see the city lights of Melbourne and the outlying coast, so I'd say I was at about 3000 ft before entering the craft. Not frightened from what I can remember, more in awe at the time. Such a wonderful experience. (Internet posting, ASP-L)

The majority of abductees, however, describe their experiences as terrifying. In her book, *How to Defend Yourself against Alien Abduction,* Ann Druffel writes:

> There are . . . various stages in the abduction process, which differ somewhat from witness to witness. Some abductees sense the approach of intruding entities before any physiological effects are noted. Usually general paralysis abruptly sets in, rendering the human being unable to move except for slight head and eye movements. Many experiencers, awakening already paralyzed, sense unseen presences around their bed. Although unseen, the presences cause overwhelming terror. Other experiencers awake already paralyzed and terrified to see the entities materialized, fully or partially. (Druffel 1998, 16)

The typical description of the "bedroom alien abduction" will by now seem quite familiar; even the strategy for escaping aliens recalls the night-mare tradition.

> Mental Struggle is an effective technique to use when the witness still feels free to use his or her mind to protest against the invasion, even though the witness is paralyzed and terrified. To describe it briefly, Mental Struggle involves sustained willpower while attempting to move some small part of the body, such as a finger or toe. When the witness succeeds in making that slight movement, the paralysis generally breaks abruptly, and the entities immediately vanish. (Druffel 1998, 21)

More than thirty years ago, Hufford noted a connection between sleep paralysis and certain types of alien abductions (1976). The accounts given by abductees or "experiencers" are believed by many to be explained by sleep paralysis (Blackmore 1994; Newman and Baumeister 1996; Randle, Estes, and Cone 1999; Rønnevig 2007). Some characteristics of alien abduction experiences, such as paralysis, terror, images of frightening intruders, and levitation, do bear a striking resemblance to the experiences reported by people who suffer from night-mares. Differences do remain, though, between sleep paralysis and certain alien abductions (particularly those that occur during the day, take place outside, and are unrelated to sleep) and for this reason some have claimed that a direct link between sleep paralysis and alien abduction experiences has yet to be firmly established (Appelle 2000). In research conducted at the University of California, Los Angeles, for example, physicists Jean-Christophe Terrillon and Sirley Marques-Bonham found that, although about half of the respondents they recruited from a sleep Web site invoked a paranormal cause to explain their nocturnal paralyses, none interpreted their experiences as alien abductions: "Either individuals who report alien abductions have chosen not to post messages, or the association between [sleep paralysis] and alien abductions is not as strong as it is generally thought" (2001, 115). A third possibility, however, is that self-identified abductees are unlikely to visit a sleep-related Web site, since they do not attribute their encounters to a parasomnia.

If we accept the assertion that a significant number of alien abduction accounts parallel night-mare experiences, what is the reason for this similarity? Psychologists Richard McNally and Susan Clancy explain that alien abduction is a "culturally available script" for night-mare sufferers.[8] As a result of representations of extraterrestrials on television and in films, few people in the United States are unaware of "what aliens look like" or how they are supposed to behave: "Why do some people come to believe that their sleep paralysis experiences . . . are caused by extraterrestrials? The answer is that their symptoms, feelings, and experiences are consistent with what they already know—or "know"—about alien abduction" (Clancy 2005, 37).[9] Clancy interviewed "approximately 50 abductees" who had been recruited through newspaper ads that read, in part: "Seeking people who may have been contacted or abducted by aliens, to participate in a memory study" (2005, 107). Describing a weekend which she subsequently spent with people who self-identified as alien abductees, Clancy wrote: "Well, this wasn't a crowd of graduate students in science. Like most people in the world they hadn't been drilled in the application of logic, argument, rigorous thinking" (2005, 28). Clancy viewed the abductees as "people who had developed memories of a traumatic event that I could be fairly certain had never occurred" (2005, 20). Later, she revealed her skepticism regarding the aliens themselves:

> Wouldn't you think these mentally and technologically superior beings would have something more interesting to do . . . than hang around North America kidnapping its more creative and intuitive inhabitants, in order to do the same experiments over and over again? Why are these genius aliens so dim? After 50 years of abducting us, why are they still taking the same bits and pieces? Don't they have freezers? (Clancy 2005, 105)

I share with Clancy a worldview that does not include current extraterrestrial visitation, but, as an anthropologist and folklorist, and in order to try to understand these phenomena from the experiencers' perspective, I undertook my research into the night-mare and, later, the mystery of the Hmong sudden nocturnal deaths, without starting from the premise that certain beliefs or interpretations of personal experiences are unfounded. This seems no more scientific than "knowing" the experience is real.[10]

Those who believe in the possibility of alien abductions disagree, equally vehemently, with the idea that sleep paralysis sufficiently explains reported experiences. John E. Mack, a psychiatrist at Harvard University Medical School, was the most prominent defender of the possibility of abductions (before his untimely death in 2004). Mack argued that sleep paralysis does not fit the evidence, noting that at least a few abduction reports come from remote places where people are not exposed to movies or other mass media tales of UFOs, and that many abductions occur in daylight and involve people who seem to have been awake and alert (Mack 1994). Some experiencers offer a different challenge, suggesting that aliens may be clever enough to use sleep paralysis as a strategy in carrying out their kidnappings: "Did you ever think that it's possible that the aliens can induce [sleep paralysis]? After all, they have to have a way to subdue their victims to begin with" (Internet posting, rebeldoctor.blogspot.com); "I have had [sleep paralysis] and I know that there are some aliens that like to do those things (grays)" (Internet posting, ASP-L).

There is clearly a connection between some sleep paralysis and some alien abduction accounts. How that connection should be interpreted, however, is less obvious. Folklorist Thomas E. Bullard studies alien abduction accounts as constituting "an unusually well-structured legend type" (1989, 147). He writes that "these accounts share many motifs with legends of supernatural encounters as otherworldly journeys, but reconcile the fantastic elements with a supposedly alien technology to settle comfortably among the rest of UFO lore" (1989, 147). Clancy asserts that "alien-abduction memories are best understood as resulting from a blend of fantasy-proneness, memory distortion, culturally available scripts, sleep hallucinations, and scientific illiteracy, aided and abetted by the suggestions and reinforcement of hypnotherapy" (Clancy 2005, 138).[11] She notes that while her subjects weren't "seriously psychologically impaired," they displayed personalities that were "particularly imaginative and prone to fantasy" (2005, 132). The abductees she spoke to "appear to have trouble with source monitoring . . . they were likely to confuse things they had thought about and imagined with things they had actually seen, read, and heard in movies, books, or TV shows" (2005, 133). In summarizing the common features of the people she interviewed, though, Clancy writes: "What can we say conclusively about this diverse group of abductees? In the end, not much" (2005, 134).

J. Allan Cheyne, a psychologist at the University of Waterloo who has done groundbreaking psychological research on the features of sleep paralysis, summarizes the relevance of the alien abduction controversy for sleep paralysis research:

> The present argument is not that accounts of UFO abductions are false memories, although it is not inconsistent with that view or with the possibility that what we have are often badly reconstructed, misinterpreted, and misattributed accounts (Clark and Loftus 1996). Rather the present view is that they are often vivid and accurate memories of real and often truly bizarre experiences for which most members of industrialized societies have no immediate and convincing conventional explanation. The experiences are entirely consistent with nocturnal assault and abduction. Many elect to deny the evidence of their senses and accept mainstream scientific explanations having to do with psychological suggestion or brain functioning. A few, however, take their experiences at face value and continue to describe their experiences in narratively rich terms with incursions of cultural elements consistent with alien abduction. (Cheyne n.d., 23)

(Re)Building Community

The lack of information that results from the absence of a shared night-mare tradition causes confusion, misdiagnosis, and suffering. In recent years, though, people who experience night-mares have turned increasingly to information technology for assistance. The Internet is playing a major role in reintroducing the night-mare to American society and providing a forum in which people who experience sleep paralysis can find, learn from, and comfort one another. (The option of anonymity is no doubt an attractive aspect of online communication.) If you search the Internet for "sleep paralysis," you will retrieve hundreds of thousands of results (527,000 hits from Google on April 21, 2010). Searching on YouTube yields 910 video results for "sleep paralysis," ranging from lectures and slide presentations to individual video logs describing personal encounters to footage of people in the throes of night-mare attacks.

One of the most active and popular sites for discussions of night-mare attacks is the Awareness during Sleep Paralysis Listserv (ASP-L). Over 900 group members regularly exchange descriptions of encounters, share advice and interpretations, and disseminate findings from recent sleep paralysis research. The following introduction greets visitors to the Web site:

> ASP, the Awareness during Sleep Paralysis list is an experience oriented forum for discussing ASP in relation to Lucid Dreams, Alien Abductions, Out of Body Experiences, Incubus/Succubus Encounters, Old Hag Attacks, Supernatural Assaults or Attacks by demonic entities and energy vampires, Psychic Attacks, and their equivalents in other cultures; sharing

experiences of Awareness during Sleep Paralysis; and supporting experiencers who might otherwise be engulfed in fear to take control of their experiences by banishing bothersome entities, resisting/preventing alien abduction, establishing a positive relationship to non-human intelligences or transforming the experience into a Lucid Dream or Out-of-Body Experience—possibly one with transforming spiritual significance. By 'Experiencer Oriented' I mean that the list is moderated to provide a safe place to share experiences. Our concern is not so much the reality status of alien beings as it is with evaluating techniques for transforming negative experiences into positive ones.

While not all list members share the paranormal/spiritual view of sleep paralysis stated on the home page, many do, and the same is true for members of other virtual communities that have formed using social media resources such as Facebook or Twitter. Although these online communities are exposed to current developments in sleep research (through informational postings and news updates), scientific knowledge about sleep paralysis has not displaced spiritual, religious, or paranormal interpretations. "Current scientific knowledge about the night-mare, and the acceptance of that knowledge, does not impede spiritual interpretations; and the discovery of a large number of other experiencers, with complex and similar subjective experiences, tends to be perceived as confirmation of the reality—that is, the nonimaginary nature—of sleep paralysis" (Hufford 2005, 30). It is unclear why or how one interpretation of a night-mare experience is favored over another. Some people understand the events as alien abductions, encounters with ancestors' spirits, or attacks by demons; others seek no explanation at all. Although the exact nature of the relationship remains unclear, the night-mare experience clearly contributes to broader cultural ideas about the spiritual and supernatural world.

2

Continuities

A Transhistorical Bestiary

"The modifications which nightmare assumes are infinite; but one passion is almost never absent—that of utter and incomparable dread."

—Robert MacNish (1834, 123)

The symptoms of the night-mare experience have been studied in relation to sleep paralysis in the last quarter century, but the night-mare spirit itself has persisted for millennia. The entity has stalked human beings throughout history, not merely within a particular society or during a specific time. In fact, the ubiquity of the night-mare led one nineteenth-century scholar to suggest that it was the origin of all mythology (Laistner 1889). Although it is difficult to imagine a researcher making this sweeping assertion today, the night-mare's prominent role in folk tradition through the ages is clear. The night-mare's past is worth exploring for what it reveals about successive eras' conceptualizations of the relationship between mind and body. Although the night-mare entity has been known by various names since ancient times, expectations regarding the physical manifestations of its uniquely evil habits have remained remarkably constant throughout its long history. We have seen that the defining features of the night-mare form a distinct and stable experience. The characteristics that shape this easily discernible pattern include the impression of wakefulness, an inability to move or speak, a realistic perception of the immediate environment, intense fear and anxiety, lying in a supine position, a feeling of pressure on the chest, difficulty breathing, and the awareness of a "presence" that is often seen or heard.

Alu

One of the earliest surviving written descriptions of the night-mare is an Assyrian reference to the evil spirit *alu*, a demon that "hides itself in dark corners and caverns in the rock, haunting ruins and deserted buildings, and slinking through the streets at night like a pariah dog" ready to rush out and envelop the unwary "as with a garment" (Thompson 1903, Tablet 1B; Thompson 1908, 81).

The *alu* creeps into its intended victim's bedroom in darkness, pouncing on the unsuspecting sleeper. There is also a Babylonian reference to "the man whom an evil *alu* hath enveloped on his bed" (Rawlinson 1861–1864, 4:50). This nightmare is a demon "which throws itself heavily on a sleeper, preventing him from moving or opening his eyes, and which disappears as soon as he awakes" (1:44). Although only fragments of these narratives remain, the features of the assault—the heavy, "enveloping" presence that oppresses sleepers and thwarts their movements—make it clear that the attacker is a night-mare.

Lilith

One of the most notorious manifestations of the night-mare entity is the female spirit Lilith. The earliest mention of a demonic being that appears to be related to Lilith is found in the Sumerian King list (circa 2400 BCE), which states that the father of the great hero Gilgamesh was a *Lillu*-demon (Patai 1990). The *Lillu* was one of four related evil spirits; the other three were *Lilitu*, a female demon (probably the prototype for the Hebrew Lilith); *Ardat Lili*, Lilith's maidservant, who had sex with men at night and then bore demonically hybrid children; and *Irdu Lili, Ardat Lili*'s male counterpart who impregnated women during his nocturnal visits (Jacobsen 1939; Stol 1993).

A Babylonian terra-cotta relief, dating from about 2000 BCE, depicts Lilith in human form—with the notable exception of her wings and owl feet. She is standing on two reclining lions and flanked by owls, indicating both her potent command and her nocturnal domain. A seventh-century BCE tablet found in northern Syria shows Lilith as a winged sphinx across whose body is written, "O, Flyer in a dark chamber,/Go away at once, O Lili!" (Patai 1990, 222). These lines are representative of texts from a genre of formulas designed to protect women in labor.

There is one brief, but nonetheless highly contested, reference to Lilith in the Torah: "Wildcats shall meet with hyenas, goat-demons shall call to each other; there too Lilith shall repose, and find a place to rest. There shall the owl nest and lay and hatch and brood in its shadow" (Isa. 34:14). Since the Hebrew term (*lilit*) used in this context is a *hapax legomenon*—a word that occurs only once in a particular text—it is impossible to make a definitive statement as to its usage and meaning. In English-language Bibles, *lilit* is occasionally translated as "screech owl"; in the Vulgate, Jerome translated the word as *lamia*, an evil being that killed infants and seduced sleeping men. Although it is not possible to identify this early *lilit* conclusively as a female night-mare spirit, the figure described is clearly associated with evil, the night, and flight.

Lilith next alights textually on the Talmud, the Jewish commentaries on the Torah (circa 400 CE). The references to her are again quite brief, but here their sketchy quality seems to indicate that there was already a firmly established cultural understanding of Lilith's wicked behavior that made explicit details and explanation unnecessary. We learn that she has wings (Nid. 24b) and long hair (Erub. 100b) and that she is, at least partially, human in appearance. Men are admonished to prevent her access to them at night: "One may not sleep in a house alone, and whoever sleeps in a house alone is seized by Lilith" (Shab. 151a; fn: "The night demon"). These limited Talmudic allusions are the first (at least in literary records) to identify Lilith as both a demon of the night and a night-mare figure.

The relatively scanty Talmudic material on Lilith is supplemented by much richer data from Aramaic inscriptions on incantation bowls. Several seventh-century CE ceramic bowls have been found which are engraved with magical texts directed against Lilith. (It seems likely that the formulas themselves originated in the oral traditions of much earlier times.) While the Talmud reflects the views of the learned elite regarding Lilith, these incantation bowls reveal her reputation in the general community. The inscriptions indicate that, during the night, female Liliths have sex with sleeping men (and male *Lilin* couple with women) in order to breed demonic offspring. Once they succeed in joining themselves to a human being, they are considered married and must be formally divorced before they can be forced to leave (Patai 1990). Women in labor and newborn babies are particularly vulnerable to attacks since Lilith is jealous of her victims' human partners. She also attempts to prevent the birth of human children by creating fertility problems or causing complications during childbirth (Scerba 1999).

In addition to instilling terror, Lilith's attacks were thought occasionally to be fatal (Chambers 1999). Lilith hates children born to human couples and attacks them, sucking their blood and strangling them while they sleep. (Her victims might themselves become assaulting demons, similar to victims of other supernatural figures, such as vampires.) In the Jewish folk tradition, circumcision protected male infants from Lilith's murderous aggression. The eight-day period following a boy's birth marked a time of escalating concern for the family, culminating in an all-night vigil to ensure that he was not attacked before the day of circumcision.

The earliest form of the most familiar version of the Lilith legend appears in *The Alphabet of Ben Sira*, an anonymous work most likely written at some point during the seventh to the eleventh centuries;[1] although, again, it is impossible to know how much earlier the story may have been present in folk and oral traditions. It is here that we find Lilith portrayed as Adam's first wife. The idea of Eve having a predecessor is not new to this text, but prior written references make no specific mention of Lilith. According to "Ben Sira,"

[God] said, 'It is not good for man to be alone' (Gen. 2:18). He then created a woman for Adam, from the earth, as He had created Adam himself, and called her Lilith. Adam and Lilith began to fight. She said, 'I will not lie below,' and he said, 'I will not lie beneath you, but only on top. For you are fit only to be in the bottom position, while I am to be in the superior one.' Lilith responded, 'We are equal to each other inasmuch as we were both created from the earth.' But they would not listen to one another. When Lilith saw this, she pronounced the Ineffable Name and flew away into the air.

God immediately sent three angels to bring her back. They came upon Lilith at sea.

They told her God's word, but she did not wish to return. The angels said, "We shall drown you in the sea." "Leave me!" she said. "I was created only to cause sickness to infants. If the infant is male, I have dominion over him for eight days after his birth, and if female, for twenty days." When the angels heard Lilith's words, they insisted she go back. But she swore to them by the name of the living and eternal God: "Whenever I see you or your names or your forms in an amulet, I will have no power over that infant." (Stern and Mirsky 1998, 183–184)

In contrast to Eve, Lilith was not created from Adam, but, like him, from the earth—she therefore considered herself his equal. Given the significance of lying supine for night-mare experiences, it is interesting that Lilith and Adam's relationship ended over a disagreement about who should assume this position.

Over the last few decades, the legend from *The Alphabet* has been the most frequently quoted in describing the origins of Lilith, although, in some instances, the details of the night-mare tradition and the references to child-killing are routinely ignored.[2] Ben Sira's biography of Lilith has rather been transformed into a feminist allegory of the prelapsarian equality of women and men. *Lilith* magazine, for example, "charts Jewish women's lives with exuberance, rigor, affection, *subversion* and style" [emphasis mine]—and the independent publication's Web site quotes the Ben Sira text as the inspiration for the magazine title.

It is remarkable that (with the exception of contemporary feminist readings of the story) the Lilith night-mare spirit has retained essentially the same form for thousands of years. Anthropologist and folklorist Raphael Patai observes that "a citizen of Sumer circa 2500 BCE and an East European Hasidic Jew in 1880 CE had very little in common as far as the higher levels of religion were concerned. But they would have readily recognized each other's beliefs about the pernicious machinations of Lilith, and each other's apotropaic measures for driving her away or escaping her enticements" (1990, 251).

Ephialtes

The male night-mare is well represented in the literature of ancient Greece, where he is typically known as *ephialtes* ("leap upon"). Because the Greeks considered being choked or strangled to be one consequence of a night-mare attack, the entity was also called *pnigalion* ("throttler"). As is the case with Assyrian and Babylonian text fragments and the early allusions to Lilith, ancient Greek writings depict a syndrome that is unmistakably that of the night-mare. The crushing pressure that the evil spirit exerts on the supine bodies of its victims remains a common theme. According to Soranos,[3] a second-century CE physician, "the sleeper feels that somebody is sitting on his chest or suddenly jumps upon it or that somebody climbs up and crushes him heavily with his weight. The sufferer feels incapacity to move, torpidity, and inability to speak. Attempts to speak often result only in single, inarticulate sounds" (Roscher 1900, 19).

Ancient Greek writings attest to the remarkable stability of the core night-mare experience over the past two millennia, but, just as we have seen in contemporary settings, specific explanations for the experience varied and competing interpretations coexisted. In opposition to the popular conception of night-mares as the visits of evil spirits, for example, the ancient Greek physicians denounced any suggestion of supernatural origins. According to Soranos, the sleeper may be convinced that the pressing demon is trying to violate him or her: "Some are so affected by empty visions that they believe they are being attacked and forced to the vilest acts" (Roscher 1900, 19). Physicians argued that the night-mare's "empty visions" found their origin not in the supernatural, but in a variety of gastric disturbances following the eating of indigestible food, general overeating, or alcoholic excess. They noted that the state of "sleep-drunkenness," the transitional phase between sleep and wakefulness, is particularly favorable to the production of night-mares. Sometimes, before falling completely asleep or just after waking up, visions of the "dream" may persist so vividly that the sleeper mistakenly believes that he or she sees the vision in actual reality. Although ancient Greek physicians associated the night-mare with epilepsy and madness, they considered it a true disease only if it occurred chronically (Roscher 1900).

Despite the development of naturalistic explanations, the popular belief in ephialtes as an actual being persisted for some time. Ephialtes was thought to be a shape-shifter, able to take on various forms during his nocturnal attacks on helpless human victims. He might initially appear as a familiar person before transforming into a horribly disfigured creature. The dead could also reappear as vengeful night-mares. The Roman poet Horace describes several witch-like hags attempting to murder an innocent boy to obtain a love charm from his "parched marrow and dried liver." The unfortunate child pleads with them to spare his life, but when he realizes that they cannot be swayed from their evil purpose, he threatens to return from the dead to attack them: "Every night, incumbent on your troubled breasts/I will chase off your sleep with fear and trembling" (Roscher 1900, 28). The revenant (ephialtes) became a well-known manifestation of the night-mare spirit, and fear-induced sleep loss was a classic consequence of an attack by such a being. Soranos explains: "Those who have suffered from the affliction for a long time are pale and thin, for, because of their fear, they do not get sleep" (Roscher 1900, 28). The gaunt, drawn appearance of the night-mare sufferer, particularly on the morning after an attack, is commonplace in folk tradition (as we have seen with the haggard/hag-ridden connection in Newfoundland).

In addition to purely terrifying attacks brought on by ephialtes, the ancient Greeks and Romans also recognized a type of sexual experience involved in supernatural contact related to sleep. Unlike Horace's vengeful revenant, ephialtes could also appear with sexual intent. The Greek historian Herodotus provides an account of an ephialtes who appeared to the (unnamed) wife of King Ariston of Sparta in the form of the king himself—although it was in actuality the spirit of the deceased hero Astrobacus. According to the queen:

> There came to me an appearance like to Ariston, and lay with me, and then put on me the garlands which he had. So when that figure was gone, presently Ariston came to me. Seeing the garlands on me, he asked me who had given them; I said they were his gift, but he denied it. Then I said, and swore it, that . . . he had come a little while ago and lain with me and so given me the garlands. When Ariston saw that I swore to that, he perceived that the hand of heaven was in the matter. (Herodotus 6, 65–69)

Although ephialtes could apparently manifest as both erotic and nonerotic night-mares, the precise differentiation that was made in the classical world between sexual sleep-related experiences and attacks of the night-mare remains difficult to determine (Hufford 1982).

Pan

The night-mare was not only a shape-shifter that could morph into a variety of forms, it could also manifest as a hideous hybrid, combining both human and animal features. Ephialtes was particularly identified with minor woodland deities, such as Pan and the satyrs (Roscher 1900). The ancient Greeks depicted these beings as primarily human from the waist up, but with goat horns and legs.[4] Pan's attacks were associated with *panikos* or panic; precisely the type of response appropriate to a night-mare attack. His visits were intimately connected with feelings of terror, and he was seen as the initiator of dreams, visions, and night-mares—particularly those that create sudden and overpowering fright.

Scholars have proposed a number of imaginative theories as they surmise how Pan came to be associated with the night-mare. The German classicist Wilhelm Roscher suggests, "The usual bedding in ancient times was the skin of a goat or cloth made of goat's hair, which by its very nature must have conjured up the appearance of goat-like nightmare demons in the person afflicted with the nightmare" (1900, 72). Literary scholar Nicolas Kiessling contends (no less fancifully) that "in the rude imagination of the sex-starved shepherd this god not unnaturally took on the shape and actions of his rams and he-goats in the mating season" (1977, 4). Despite these conjectures, however, there is no evidence that the night-mare of antiquity had a central erotic component. Roscher, who traced the night-mare from ancient Greece through the Renaissance in a work entitled *Pan and the Nightmare* (1900), took for granted the existence of a night-mare/erotic dream complex already in classical antiquity, but there is no indication that Pan night-mares possessed an erotic dimension until the second-century CE dream interpreter Artemidorus (author of *Oneirocritica*, a dream interpretation manual) wrote:

> Ephialtes is identified with Pan but he has a different meaning. If he oppresses or weighs a man down without speaking, it signifies tribulations and distress. But whatever he says upon interrogation is true. If he gives someone something or has sexual intercourse with someone, it foretells great profit, especially if he does not weigh that person down. (Artemidorus 1975, 2:37)

Before this time, folk tradition apparently maintained two relatively distinct categories of sleep-related experience: the erotic interaction and the pressing night-mare attack (Chambers 1999).

Unclassifiable Entities

Before I present the history and evolution of other discrete night-mare beings, I want to emphasize that not all encounters (or more accurately, not all descriptions of encounters) lend themselves to such ready categorization. There may have been many more examples of night-mares in the world's historical traditions that were simply not preserved in sufficient detail. One well-known instance for which there is inadequate narrative information is the biblical description of Jacob's nocturnal wrestling with a "stranger" (Gen. 32:25). The potential allusion to a night-mare is intriguing, perhaps, but despite ongoing debates among those interested in the history of parasomnias—that is, undesirable sleep-related phenomena—there is not enough information to be able to classify the struggle as a night-mare encounter. The same is true for the account of a mystical experience of the Prophet Muhammad. Some details of the event sound quite familiar, but the interaction cannot be definitively categorized. One night in 610 CE, Muhammad was awakened from sleep and felt himself "enveloped by a devastating divine presence."

> An angel had appeared to him and given him a curt command: 'Recite!' (*iqra!*) . . . Muhammad refused, protesting, "I am not a reciter!" [that is, he was not one of the ecstatic soothsayers claiming to recite inspired oracles]. But . . . the angel simply enveloped him in an overpowering embrace, so that he felt as if all the breath was being squeezed from his body. Just as he felt he could bear it no longer, the angel released him and again commanded him to "Recite!" (*iqra!*). Again Muhammad refused and again the angel embraced him until he felt that he had reached the limits of his endurance. Finally, at the end of a third terrifying embrace Muhammad found the first words of a new scripture [ultimately called the *Qur'an* or Recitation] pouring from his mouth. (Armstrong 1994, 137)

In the account of Muhammad's struggle, some characteristics of the night-mare are evident, including awakening to a presence, hearing a brief audible command, and being held in a crushing embrace.

The night-mare figure is clearly evident in later Muslim folk traditions. Avicenna (Ibn Sina), one of the greatest medieval physicians, describes the night-mare in his *Canon*, using three Arabic terms: *al-kabus*, the squeezer; *al-khanaq*, the strangler; and *al-gathum*, that which alights or perches (Jarcho 1980, 254). (Like the ancient Greek physicians, Avicenna believed that the night-mare was related to disturbances of the brain: apoplexy, epilepsy, or mania.) The fact that there is evidence of subsequent folk traditions, however, is insufficient grounds on which to characterize either Jacob's or Muhammad's encounters as a night-mare, particularly in the absence of more detailed descriptions of the phenomenology of their experiences.

Mara/Mare

The night-mare not only thrived in ancient and classical traditions, but in Anglo-Saxon and Old Norse beliefs, as well. According to Ernest Jones, the Welsh neurologist and psychoanalyst, "*mara*, from the verb *merran*, literally means a 'crusher,' and the connotation of a crushing weight on the breast is common to the corresponding words in allied languages (Icelandic *mara*, Danish *mare*, Low German *moore*, Bohemian *mara*, Swedish *mara*, Old High German *mara*)" (1931, 243). The mara is referenced in the earliest Anglo-Saxon literature, in the epic poem *Beowulf*. The monster Grendel, referred to at least twice by the term *maere*, is described as a descendent of Cain (Kiessling 1968). (Early mystical Jewish literature depicts Lilith as returning to torment Adam after her sojourn in the Red Sea, but not before attacking Cain and bearing numerous spirits and demons as a result of their union.) Grendel, a cannibalistic devourer, invariably carries out his attacks in the dead of night on sleeping men, crushing and tearing them apart. Prior to Beowulf's confrontation with Grendel, Hrothgar explains that previous heroes have been defeated, in part, because they were unable to remain awake during the night when Grendel preferred to attack.

The mara makes another literary appearance in the twelfth-century Icelandic poem, *Heimskringla*. In some societies, the night-mare is not attributed to an evil spirit, but rather to the magical activities of living beings who are motivated by envy and malice. The Finnish princess, Driva, was angered because her husband, Vanlandi, left her to visit Sweden for several years. When Vanlandi did not come home by the time he had promised, Driva bribed a witch to enchant Vanlandi into returning or, if the sorcery failed, to kill him. When Vanlandi's companions would not allow him to leave, the witch crushed the warrior to death.

> A drowsiness overcame him and he lay down to sleep. But he had hardly gone to sleep when he called out, saying that a nightmare rode him. His men went to him and wanted to help him. But when they took hold of his head the nightmare trod on his legs so they nearly broke; and when they seized his feet it pressed down on his head so that he died. (Sturluson 1932, 9–10)

The Swedes cremated Vanlandi's body near the Skuta River and set a stone for him which read: "There trod the troll-wise sorceress on the warrior lord. And there was burned on the Skuta bank that generous man whom the Mare killed" (Sturluson 1932, 10). This medieval Icelandic example not only blurs the distinction between the mara and the human witch, but incorporates the belief, as seen in the Lilith tradition, that the night-mare can cause death.

British historian Owen Davies argues that by the early modern period, the archaic mara was no longer a current concept in many countries, including France and England, and that the principal figure of supernatural evil in most people's lives was the witch. Even in regions where belief in the mara continued, it was closely linked with a living, human witch. In Poland, the term *zmora* designated "people who are alive and able to disturb their neighbors' sleep by making them feel an enormous weight resting upon their body" (Schiffman 1987). As we will see, this association of the night-mare with human witches became one of the most salient historical transformations of the pressing spirit in early modern Europe.

Incubus and Succubus

The term *incubus* (from the Latin *incubare*, which means "to lie upon") came into use around the beginning of the Common Era (Stewart 2002). Several centuries later, *succubus* ("to lie under") became the word reserved to denote the female pressing spirit. The feminine term is conceptually confusing, though, because the succubus typically lies *upon* the sleeper, as well. More recently, the gender distinction has become blurred and *incubus* has been used to refer to night-mare spirits of either sex.

Since ancient times, people recognized that at least two different kinds of experience were included in traditions of supernatural contact related to sleep: one that primarily involved feelings of terror and another that contained a sex-ual element (Chambers 1999). Some terms for these events have been used in a restricted sense, referring to sexual encounters or to terrifying attacks involving pressure and restraint. Other terms are broader and can refer to either or both experiences. *Incubus* appears to have had sexual connotations from its initial appearance in early Christian tradition.

Monks of the early Church believed that demons inspired sexual dreams. These evil spirits were able to manipulate individuals' thoughts and memories and to activate or set in motion sinful ideas. Unholy thoughts were thus origi-nally conceptualized as an inevitable part of the human condition. According to Evagrius, who became a monk in Egypt around 382 CE, "it is not up to us whether evil thoughts might trouble the soul or leave it in peace. What does depend on us is whether they linger or not, and whether they set the passions in motion or not" (Stewart 2002, 289). A sleeper, for example, had some degree of power in determining to what extent he would be affected by his dreams. If sleep events were thus controllable, then anyone who experienced an unholy dream was potentially responsible. The culpability of human beings was of particular con-cern in determining the level of sinfulness involved in erotic dreams and noc-turnal emissions. Excusable nocturnal emissions were thought to become sinful if they resulted from erotic dreams that the sleeper had allowed to linger, and, most importantly, had been consensual (Elliott 1999, 20). The Christian laity thus came to view the erotic dream as dangerous.[5] Potentially pleasurable sexual dreams were demonized and joined with manifestations of the pressing, stran-gling night-mare to give rise to a night-mare/erotic dream complex. The avail-able label adopted to refer to this dual experience was *incubus*. The sexual night-mare and the terrorizing night-mare traditions were therefore not merged until the early Christian period, when the "control of inner cupidity became a salient diagnostic of spiritual progress" (Stewart 2002, 280).

It was not only the Christian laity who recognized the incubus; Augustine writes in *De Civitate Dei* that he accepts the reality of the existence of these evil erotic beings.

> There is, too, a very general rumor, which many have verified by their
> own experience, or which trustworthy persons who have heard the expe-
> rience of others corroborate, that sylvans and Pans, who are commonly

called "incubi," had often made wicked assaults upon women, and satisfied their lust upon them; and that certain devils, called Duses by the
Gauls, are constantly attempting and effecting this impurity is so generally affirmed, that it were impudent to deny it. (Augustine 15:23)

As we have seen in the context of the contemporary night-mare, however,
this eroticization of the encounter is not a peculiarity of European history. The
erotic form of the night-mare tradition is less easily traced than its primary features, but it is an aspect of the experience that appears in different historical
and cultural contexts.[6]

Witch Trials

In the sixteenth century, by the time of the Protestant and Catholic
Reformations, the witch hunts had already begun. Trials often included accusations of sex with the devil, and the incubus was not infrequently a key figure in
the legal proceedings. The primary charge against women accused of witchcraft
was that they had made a pact with Satan; sexual encounters with the devil were
believed to seal the pact, as well as confer on the devil complete power over the
witch. The allegation that a human being had had sex with the devil (in the
form of an incubus) was, in fact, the chief accusation in many trials, and countless women were burned as witches as a direct result of this particular interpretation of a night-mare attack (Powell 1973). Part of the debate surrounding
witchcraft focused on whether submission to an incubus was sufficient evidence that a woman was a witch. This question contributed to a larger controversy over whether witchcraft genuinely involved unnatural acts or whether its
primary crime was heresy (Hufford 1982).

Manuals devoted to witch hunting developed detailed schema of incubi
and succubi that interacted with human beings to further the devil's cause. The
most notorious of these compendia of lore about witches, incubi, and demons
in the later Middle Ages is *Malleus Maleficarum* (1487), written by two Dominican
friars, Heinrich Kramer and Jakob Sprenger. The 1495 edition of the text opens
with Pope Innocent VIII's famous "Witch Bull": "It has indeed lately come to Our
ears, not without afflicting Us with bitter sorrow, that . . . many persons of both
sexes, unmindful of their own salvation and straying from the Catholic Faith,
have abandoned themselves to devils, incubi, and succubi." Kramer and Sprenger
give particularly forceful expression to the traditional incubus beliefs. The authors
contend that women are more susceptible to the night-mare than men—since
they are more feeble and credulous and less self-controlled—and that widows
and virgins (particularly nuns) are disturbed more often than married women.
In a change from earlier views, Kramer and Sprenger also note that "the Incubus
devils used to infest women against their wills," but in the present, witches
"willingly embrace this most foul and miserable servitude" (1971, 111).

Incubi were believed to be incapable of procreating without the assistance of human beings. Kramer and Sprenger describe the elaborate process whereby a succubus gathers semen by having intercourse with a man and then transforming herself, or transmitting the semen, to an incubus, who in turn impregnates a woman. The authors devote much of their text to the habits of incubi and succubi and discuss a number of questions, such as "How do witches copulate with incubi?" and "Does the incubus operate more at one time than another?" Literary historian Nicolas Kiessling points out that the authors of *Malleus Maleficarum* "marshal lengthy arguments from every church father that they have available and every word of Scripture that has been related to the subject. Their reason and logic show little imagination. But they are utterly frank in describing the lurid details of intercourse with demons" (1977, 38). The effect of the exhaustive witchcraft manuals, as well as the prosecutions, was to further elaborate upon and maximally diffuse the night-mare tradition.

Contemporary historians and folklorists have noted that it is possible, even likely, that many of the preternatural experiences described during witch trials did not initially contain sexual elements (e.g., Chambers 1999). Rather, inquiring authorities assumed that witchcraft must involve sexual acts with the devil/incubus and so they steered narratives in that direction through their questioning: "Judges showed a particular interest in the issue of whether the intercourse with the devil was voluntary or forced, frightening or pleasurable. Whether or not actual erotic nightmares or erotic dreams had occurred to the accused, there was a likelihood that erotic nightmare scenarios would occupy a conspicuous place in the final confession" (Stewart 2002, 293). Ironically, the Church's zealous efforts to throw off the incubus appear only to have strengthened its hold.[7]

One of the best ways to study the night-mare beliefs of early modern Europe is to examine trial records of the time (Davies 2003). In England in 1599, for example, a woman named Olive Barthram was prosecuted for witchcraft. During the trial, her neighbor, Joan Jorden, testified that a shape-changing spirit sent by Barthram tormented her at night. The intruder, which entered through the chimney, was "a thick dark substance about a foot high, like to a sugar loaf, white on top."[8] On another occasion, the spirit appeared in the shape of a cat and made rustling noises:

> At 11 o'clock at night, first scraping on the walls, then knocking, after that shuffling in the rushes: ... [he] kissed her three or four times, and slavered on her, and lying on her breast he pressed her so sore that she could not speak, at other times he held her hands that she could not stir, and restrained her voice that she could not answer. (Ewen 1933, 188)

The records from the Salem witchcraft trials of 1692 reveal that the incubus played a similarly significant role in colonial American prosecutions. Cotton

Mather, a socially and politically influential Puritan minister, successfully argued that it was appropriate to admit spectral evidence into the legal proceedings (Mather 1692). Thus, in Salem, just as in the earlier trials in Europe, testimony that the accused witch's spirit (specter) appeared to the witness in a dream or vision—regardless of the physical location of the accused at the time—could be admitted as evidence.

Two of the clearest examples of these spectral night-mare encounters appear in testimony during the trials of Bridget Bishop and Susanna Martin. The transcripts of the proceedings show that during the course of Bishop's trial, Richard Coman alleged that, while he was in bed eight years before, "the curtains at the foot of the bed opened where [he] did see her and [she] presently came and lay upon [his] breast or body and so oppressed him that he could not speak nor stir, no, not so much as to awake his wife, although he endeavored much so to do it"[9] (Boyer and Nissenbaum 1977, 1:102). Similarly, during Susanna Martin's trial, Bernard Peach testified that

> being in bed on a Lord's day night he heard a scratching at the window. He saw Susanna Martin, wife of George Martin of Amsbury, come in at the window and jump down upon the floor. . . . She . . . took hold of [his feet] and drew up his body into a heap and lay upon him about an hour and a half or two hours, in all which time this deponent could not stir nor speak. Feeling himself beginning to be loosened or lightened, he began to strive to put out his hand among the clothes and took hold of her hand and brought it up to his mouth and bit three of the fingers . . . to the breaking of the bones, after which Susanna Martin went out of the chamber. (Boyer and Nissenbaum 1977, 2:562)

The transcripts of the Salem witch trials preserve such detailed accounts of night-mare episodes that we can, once again, easily recognize the consistent features of the experience. As further evidence of the stability of the night-mare's symptoms, folklorist Patricia Rickels published a small collection of night-mare accounts in 1961 from her fieldwork in Louisiana. She describes the reaction of a study participant: "I read her the account of one of Bridget Bishop's victims, written down in Salem, in 1693, and she approved it as 'Just right'" (1961, 59). Nearly three hundred years after they were first described, details of night-mare attacks were both recognizable and deemed accurate.

The question of the reality of witchcraft and the locus of responsibility for night-mare encounters was never uniformly decided during the sixteenth and seventeenth centuries, the main period of witch hunting. The belief in seductive incubi and succubi was, however, seriously challenged in the writings of Reginald Scot, who, in the process of proving that witches do not exist, dismissed all stories of evil night-mare spirits: "Thus are lecheries covered with the cloke of *Incubus* and witchcraft . . . speciallie to excuse and meinteine the knaveries and lecheries of idle priests and bawdie monkes; and to cover the shame of their lovers and concubines" (1584, 48). Scot believed that incubus accounts were fabricated to disguise the lechery of priests. He cites lines from *Canterbury Tales* to support his argument:

> Wommen may go now saufly up and doun;
> In every bussh or under every tree
> Ther is noon oother incubus but he,
> And he ne wol doun hem but dishonour. (Chaucer 1957, 3:878–881)

Thus, in "The Wife of Bath's Tale," Chaucer writes satirically that incubi became less frequent with the introduction of mendicant friars, who, he insinuates, replaced them. He asserts that "dishonoring" (in the sense of violating chastity) is well within the capability of friars—there is no need to attribute the behavior to incubi.

Another sixteenth-century work, *Daemonologie*, by King James I of England, also questions the belief in demonic incubi (although not that in witches). James uses the literary device of a debate between two fictitious characters to discuss the reality of witchcraft and, in the process, challenge the supernatural status of the incubus:

PHILOMATHES: Is it not the thing which we cal the Mare, which takes folkes sleeping in their bedds, a kinde of these spirites, whereof ye are speaking?

EPISTEMON: No, that is but a naturall sicknes, which the Mediciners hath given that name of Incubus unto ab incubando, because it being a thick fleume, falling into our breast upon the harte, while we are sleeping, intercludes so our vitall spirites, and takes all power from us, as maks us think that there were some unnaturall burden or spirite, lying upon us and holding us downe. (James I 2008, 64)

Despite growing acceptance of natural causation for the incubus, however, spectral evidence of bewitchment was accepted by courts until the eighteenth century (and beyond, in some parts of Europe) (Davies 1996). The witchcraft prosecutions continued even though there was a high degree of controversy about the status of both witches and incubus encounters. Part of the reason for this seeming inconsistency is the fact that not all instances of unusual occurrences were attributed to supernatural causes. Even a robust tradition of night-mare attacks did not preclude some events from being interpreted as figments of the imagination. As Owen Davies explains this critical difference, it was only when "the nightmare experience tied in with other misfortunes, or occurred repeatedly, that witchcraft came to be suspected or confirmed" (2003, 188).

Night-mare

In early modern times, the incubus was a standard feature of European medical treatises and the subject of occasional theses. The night-mare was secularized and naturalized, de-emphasizing the origins of its etymological root—*mara*, the pressing spirit—and the term *incubus* came to denote a set of physical symptoms rather than a supernatural entity. Between 1650 and 1850, physicians wrote more than twenty five treatises on the night-mare (Jones 1931). These medical works depicted the experience as having an entirely natural etiology. For many people, the erotic night-mare reverted to a separate experience, distinct from an encounter characterized by feelings of overwhelming fear and oppression.

British medical texts from the Enlightenment characterized the night-mare primarily in terms of its accompanying feelings of anxiety, terror, and suffocation. Three of these accounts are worth quoting at length for the evidence they provide of the historical continuity of the encounter, even in the absence of a unifying supernatural framework. Of the many authors who wrote on the subject, the overwhelming majority were themselves night-mare sufferers (as is still the case today). One of these was a Scottish physician, John Bond, who authored the first medical night-mare treatise written in English, *An Essay on the Incubus, or Night-mare* (see illustration 2.1). (Bond's treatise was based on his doctoral thesis [1751]. Although his similarly themed dissertation predates my own by close to two hundred and fifty years, I have always felt an affinity for his work.) In the book's preface, Bond discloses his personal stake in the topic as well as reports on the then-current state of night-mare research:

> Being much afflicted with the Night-mare, self-preservation made me particularly inquisitive about it. . . . The few Authors who have mention'd it . . . have also given imperfect accounts of it; which are probably owing to their not having felt it themselves: for, as it only seizes People in sleep, continues but a short time, and vanishes as soon as they awake, the Physician has not an opportunity of making observations of his own, but must take all from the description of others, who have labour'd under it. These, I believe, are the reasons that the principal Writers in Physic have taken so little notice of it. These omissions however render an inquiry into the nature of this Disease the more interesting and necessary, and, at the same time, the more difficult. (1753, preface)

He also includes the following vivid description of the experience itself:

> The Night-mare generally seizes people sleeping on their backs, and often begins with frightful dreams, which are soon succeeded by a difficult respiration, a violent oppression on the breast, and a total privation of voluntary motion. In this agony they sigh, groan, utter indistinct sounds, and remain in the jaws of death, till, by the utmost efforts of their

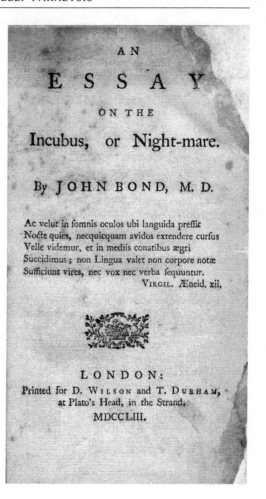

A N

E S S A Y

ON THE

Incubus, or Night-mare.

By JOHN BOND, M. D.

Ac velut in fomnis oculos ubi languida preffit
Nocte quies, necquicquam avidos extendere curfus
Velle videmur, et in mediis conatibus ægri
Succidimus; non Lingua valet non corpore notæ
Sufficiunt vires, nec vox nec verba fequuntur.
            VIRGIL. Æneid. xii,

LONDON:

Printed for D. WILSON and T. DURHAM,
at Plato's Head, in the Strand.
MDCCLIII.

2.1. Title Page of John Bond's 1753 *An Essay on the Incubus, or Night-mare.*

The treatise, which is a translation and expansion of Bond's dissertation, *De Incubo*, appears to be the first English medical work on the night-mare. The Latin text reads: "and as in dreams of night, when languorous sleep has weighed down our eyes, we seem to strive vainly to press on our eager course, and in mid effort sink helpless: our tongue lacks power, our wonted strength fails our limbs, nor voice nor words ensue" (Virgil, *Aeneid* 12.908–911). The reproduction was made from an original in the Boston Medical Library in the Francis A. Countway Library of Medicine.

nature, or some external assistance, they escape out of that dreadful torpid state. As soon as they shake off that vast oppression, and are able to move the body, they are affected by strong palpitation, great anxiety, languor, and uneasiness; which symptoms gradually abate, and are succeeded by the pleasing reflection of having escaped such imminent danger. (Bond 1753, 2–3)

Despite their literary tone, accounts such as this—related by people with firsthand experience—provide a realistic sense of the monumental terror of the night-mare. Bond's naturalistic framework for understanding the night-mare does not reduce its terror for him. He writes that he was "so much oppress'd by this enemy of rest" that "I would have given ten thousand worlds like this for some Person that would either pinch, shake, or turn me off my Back;

and I have been so much afraid of its intolerable insults, that I have slept in a chair all night, rather than give it an opportunity of attacking me in an horizontal position" (Bond 1753, 71).[10] Bond associates the night-mare with over-consumption and immoderate behavior; it is nothing but "the offspring of excess" (1753, preface). Failure to "cure" night-mares could prove fatal, but Bond asserts that the night-mare can be treated: "the most effectual remedy is to rouse them as soon as possible, by changing the position of the Body, and applying some keen stimulus immediately, such as pricking with a pin, speaking loud, etc." (71).

Medical interest in the night-mare phenomenon continued through the nineteenth century (Dacome 2004). The emphasis remained on the devastating terror that was naturally induced by the attacks. John Waller, a surgeon in England's Royal Navy—and a night-mare sufferer—attempted to elucidate the experience in order to minimize the distress of those similarly afflicted. He explains that the sleeper

> feels to be oppressed with some weight which confines him upon his back and prevents his breathing, which is now become extremely laborious, so that the lungs cannot be fully inflated by any effort he can make. The sensation is now the most painful that can be conceived; the person becomes every instant more awake and conscious of his situation: he makes violent efforts to move his limbs, especially his arms, with a view of throwing off the incumbent weight, but not a muscle will obey the impulse of the will: he groans aloud, if he has strength to do it, while every effort he makes seems to exhaust the little remaining vigour. The difficulty of breathing goes on increasing, so that every breath he draws, seems to be almost the last that he is likely to draw; the heart generally moves with increased velocity, sometimes is affected with palpitation; the countenance appears ghastly, and the eyes are half open. (1816, 22–23)

Waller's treatise also emphasizes the natural causes of the phenomenon and is memorable for his statement that, while on duty in the West Indies, he could produce an attack of incubus at any time by eating avocados (1816, 105). Waller, like Bond before him, continues the line of reasoning, evident since ancient times, that blames "indigestible foods" for night-mare attacks. This approach maintains that night-mares are the manifestation of a disordered body (due to intemperance), rather than the result of a spiritual force. A decade after Waller's publication, physician James Thatcher listed other popular natural etiologies in *American Modern Practice*: the night-mare is "a nervous affection, and arises chiefly from indigestion and oppression of the stomach, in consequence of eating a heavy supper just before going to bed. Wind in the stomach is also a very frequent cause of this complaint. Deep thought, anxiety, and a sedentary life may produce the night-mare" (Thatcher 1826, 610). Naturalistic beliefs such as these remain current today.

The final nineteenth-century medical description I will include was written by the physician Robert MacNish in *The Philosophy of Sleep*:

> Imagination cannot conceive the horrors [the night-mare] frequently gives rise to, or language describe it in adequate terms. . . . Everything horrible, disgusting or terrifying in the physical or moral world is brought before [the victim] in fearful array; he is hissed at by serpents, tortured by demons, stunned by the hollow voices and cold touch of apparitions. . . . At one moment he may have the consciousness of the malignant being at his side . . . its icy breath is felt diffusing itself over his visage, and he knows he is face-to-face with a fiend. . . . Or, he may have the idea of a monstrous hag squatted upon his breast—mute, motionless and malignant . . . whose intolerable weight crushes the breath out of his body. (1834, 123–124)

MacNish recognized that people can be fully conscious during the experience but paralyzed and mute—though sometimes they are able to produce moaning or groaning sounds. Attempting to cry out, a person may hallucinate that he or she is actually shouting and wonder "that the household are not alarmed by his noise" (1834, 126). The inhibition of speech is described clearly: "his voice is half-choked by impending suffocation, and . . . any exertion of it, farther than a deep sigh or groan, is impossible" (126). Noting that, during a night-mare, the individual is "more or less awake," MacNish describes the accompanying sense of terror as so great that the experience of it is "one of the most distressing to which human nature is subject" (123).

While the night-mare was thus subjected to the medical gaze, it managed once more to excite the supernatural imagination by leaping into the realm of art and fiction. We have already seen that the theological elaboration of the erotic night-mare reanimated the belief that the partner in a sexual dream was an actual being. Now again, when medicine had almost completely vanquished the demonic night-mare, "the romantics revitalized it in a sort of backlash against the tyranny of reason" (Stewart 2002, 300).

A mid-eighteenth-century painting, *The Nightmare*, was an enormously influential inspiration to writers and artists. More than fifty-five thousand people attended the London exhibition of the work (out of a city population totaling fewer than seven hundred and fifty thousand) (McNamara 2008). The artist, Henry Fuseli, first exhibited his painting at the Royal Academy, where it prompted reactions of shock and fascination.[11] (The 1751 version is reproduced on the cover of this book.) *The Nightmare* depicts a supine, possibly sleeping woman whose head and arms hang over the edge of a bed as she is assaulted by a demonic creature who squats heavily on her stomach. A horse head with wildly staring eyes peers through curtains in the background, and a bedside table holds a mirror that does not reflect the demon's image (Baumann, Lentzsch, Regard, and Bassetti 2007). (The equine figure is most likely a consequence of the common misconception that night-*mare* is etymologically related to a female horse.) There is no record of Fuseli's inspiration for this subject (it is also the focus of some of his other paintings), but, perhaps, as is the case with so many writers and scientists who engage the night-mare, he himself suffered from sleep paralysis.[12] Regardless of the immediate source of Fuseli's image, it "impressed itself so firmly on the mind of the public that caricaturists were immediately able to make use of it for personal or political satires, and went on using it for decades afterwards" (Powell 1973, 17) (see illustration 2.2).

Artistic representations of the night-mare in seventeenth- and eighteenth-century England often featured a female victim. The reason for this may be that the supine position was viewed as too passive for men. Consider, for example, Mercutio's joking comment in Shakespeare's *Romeo and Juliet*: "This is the hag, when maids lie on their backs,/That presses them, and learns them first to bear,/Making them women of good carriage" (I.iv.97–99). The image of the passive female night-mare victim is captured by Erasmus Darwin (a physician,

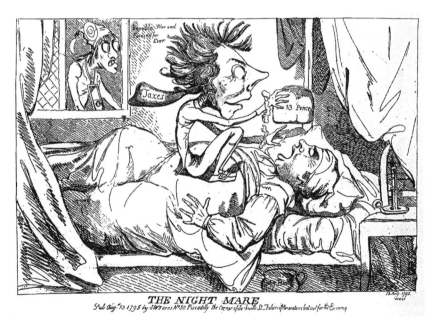

2.2. "The Night Mare" shows John Bull in bed, William Pitt as the incubus, and a French Jacobin looking through the window in place of Fuseli's horse. (Caricature of William Pitt. Attributed to Temple Webb, August 13, 1795. London, British Museum.)

naturalist, and poet, as well as the grandfather of Charles) in a poem inspired by Fuseli's painting:

> The Night-mare . . .
> Seeks some love-wilder'd Maid with sleep oppress'd,
> Alights, and grinning sits upon her breast . . .
> Back o'er her pillow sinks her blushing head,
> Her snow-white limbs hang helpless from the bed;
> While with quick sighs and suffocative breath
> Her interrupted heart-pulse swims in death . . .
> O'er her fair limbs convulsive tremors fleet;
> Start in her hands, and struggle in her feet;
> In vain to scream with quivering lips she tries,
> And strains in palsy'd lids her tremulous eyes;
> In vain she *wills* to run, fly, swim, walk, creep;
> The WILL presides not in the bower of SLEEP.
> (1791, lines 53–74)

Fuseli's painting also influenced a much better known literary work, Mary Shelley's *Frankenstein*.[13] Shelley was familiar with the painting, and her description of the dead Elizabeth appears to be modeled on Fuseli's depiction: "She was there, lifeless and inanimate, thrown across the bed, her head hanging down, and her pale and distorted features half covered by her hair" (Shelley 1831). In the introduction to the 1831 edition of *Frankenstein*, Shelley writes that her inspiration for the book came while she was vacationing in Switzerland with an illustrious group that included Lord Byron and her soon-to-be husband, Percy. In order to stave off the boredom of being confined indoors because of stormy weather, the group decided to compose horror stories.[14] Shelley was unable to come up with an idea until, late one night, she experienced what she called a "waking dream," elements of which resemble a nightmare experience:

> When I placed my head on my pillow, I did not sleep, nor could I be said to think. My imagination, unbidden, possessed and guided me, gifting the successive images that arose in my mind with a vividness far beyond the usual bounds of reverie. . . . I see them still; the very room, the dark parquet, the closed shutters, with the moonlight struggling through. . . . I could not so easily get rid of my hideous phantom; still it haunted me. I must try to think of something else. I recurred to my ghost story,—my tiresome unlucky ghost story! O! if I could only contrive one which would frighten my reader as I myself had been frightened that night! Swift as light and as cheering was the idea that broke in upon me. I have found it!

What terrified me will terrify others; and I need only describe the spectre which had haunted my midnight pillow. On the morrow I announced that I had thought of a story. I began that day with the words, It was on a dreary night of November, making only a transcript of the grim terrors of my waking dream. (Shelley 1831, 9)

Despite the view of one late nineteenth-century scholar that the "subject . . . is of such gross and revolting a nature that it should willingly be passed over in silence" (Spalding 1880, 118), there were a number of night-mare sightings in contemporary fiction. The night-mare made a variety of appearances in literary works, from a simile in Robert Louis Stevenson's *Kidnapped*—"There was that tightness on my chest that I could hardly breathe; the thought of the two men I had shot sat upon me like a nightmare" (Stevenson 1886, 92)—to a leading role in Thomas Hardy's *Wessex Tales*:

Rhoda Brook dreamed—since her assertion that she really saw, before falling asleep, was not to be believed—that the young wife, in the pale silk dress and white bonnet, but with features shockingly distorted, and wrinkled as by age, was sitting upon her chest as she lay. The pressure of Mrs. Lodge's person grew heavier; the blue eyes peered cruelly into her face; and then the figure thrust forward its left hand mockingly, so as to make the wedding-ring it wore glitter in Rhoda's eyes. Maddened mentally, and nearly suffocated by pressure, the sleeper struggled; the incubus, still regarding her, withdrew to the foot of the bed, only, however, to come forward by degrees, resume her seat, and flash her left hand as before. (Hardy 1896, 73)

Efforts at night-mare spotting yield results in American literature, as well. Edgar Allan Poe's "The Fall of the House of Usher" includes a reference to Fuseli's art, as well as this passage recounted by the short story's unnamed, increasingly unsettled narrator:

Sleep came not near my couch—while the hours waned and waned away. I struggled to reason off the nervousness which had dominion over me. I endeavored to believe that much, if not all of what I felt, was due to the bewildering influence of the gloomy furniture of the room—of the dark and tattered draperies, which, tortured into motion by the breath of a rising tempest, swayed fitfully to and fro upon the walls, and rustled uneasily about the decorations of the bed. But my efforts were fruitless. An irrepressible tremor gradually pervaded my frame; and, at length, there sat upon my very heart an incubus of utterly causeless alarm. Shaking this off with a gasp and a struggle, I uplifted myself upon the pillows. (Poe 1845, 77)

A few years later, Herman Melville's description of sleep paralysis was articulated through Ishmael in *Moby Dick*:

> Slowly waking from it—half steeped in dreams—I opened my eyes and the
> before sunlit room was now wrapped in outer darkness. Instantly I felt a
> shock running through all my frame; nothing was to be seen and nothing
> was to be heard; but a supernatural hand seemed placed in mine. My arm
> hung over the counterpane, and the nameless, unimaginable silent form
> or phantom, to which the hand belonged, seemed closely seated by my
> bedside. For what seemed ages piled on ages, I lay there, frozen with the
> most awful fears, not daring to drag away my hand; yet ever thinking that
> if I could but stir it one single inch, the horrid spell would be broken.
> (Melville 1851, 31)

There is also an extended description of a night-mare in F. Scott Fitzgerald's *The
Beautiful and Damned* and an allusion in Ernest Hemingway's *The Snows of
Kilimanjaro*.

The night-mare is not restricted to fiction, however, but also appears in
other works.[15] In describing the constraints of history-making, Karl Marx writes
that the "tradition of all the generations weighs like a nightmare on the brain
of the living" (Marx 1852, 289). Marx's simile retains the sense of oppressive
weight, but in the late nineteenth century, the term *night-mare* had already
begun a process of gradual generalization, first referring to "any bad dream,"
and then "a frightening experience or thing" (Oxford English Dictionary 1989).
Over the last century, the term has been slowly drained of its original meaning.
Memories of the ancient encounters have all but faded and the narratives are
now rarely discussed. North Americans, with very few exceptions, are no longer
familiar with names for the night-mare spirit. In 1997, the *New York Times*
reported:

> Since last year, Reebok has been selling a women's running shoe dubbed
> the "Incubus." Trouble was, as an Arizona newspaper reader pointed out,
> an incubus is an evil spirit that in medieval times was thought to prey on
> sleeping women, having sex with them. A red-faced Reebok asked retail-
> ers to black out the name on the shoe boxes; the name fortunately does
> not appear on the shoe. (Vickers 1997)

More than 50,000 pairs of shoes were sold over the period of a year before
someone realized that a demon that attacked women in their sleep was a poor
choice of namesake for women's athletic apparel. Instead of disappearing along
with the night-mare's original denotation, however, episodes of nocturnal
assault have persisted. Despite the fact that the night-mare experience can no
longer be easily described in some contemporary contexts, there continue to be
encounters in widely scattered cultural settings around the world.

3

The Night-mare on the Analyst's Couch

"For the true significance of the Nightmare to be properly appreciated, first by the learned professions and then by the general public, would . . . entail consequences, both scientific and social, to which the term momentous might well be applied."

–Ernest Jones (1931, 8)

In 1887, Guy de Maupassant published "Le Horla," a tale of horror that reveals its protagonist's increasingly anguished thoughts about a nocturnal visitor through a series of diary entries:

> May 25. As the evening comes on, an incomprehensible feeling of disquietude seizes me, just as if night concealed some terrible menace toward me. I dine quickly, and then try to read, but I do not understand the words, and can scarcely distinguish the letters. Then I walk up and down my drawing-room, oppressed by a feeling of confused and irresistible fear, a fear of sleep. . . . Then, I go to bed, and I wait for sleep as a man might wait for the executioner. . . . I sleep—a long time—two or three hours perhaps—then a dream—no—a nightmare lays hold of me. I feel that I am in bed and asleep—I feel it and I know it—and I feel also that somebody is coming close to me, is looking at me, touching me, is getting on to my bed, is kneeling on my chest, is taking my neck between his hands and squeezing it—squeezing it with all his might in order to strangle me. I struggle, bound by that terrible powerlessness which paralyzes us in our dreams; I try to cry out—but I cannot; I want to move—I cannot; I try, with the most violent efforts and out of breath, to turn over and throw off this being which is crushing and suffocating me—I cannot! And then suddenly I wake up, shaken and bathed in perspiration; I light a candle and find that I am alone. (Maupassant, 4–5)

The narrator thus senses the unearthly presence of the Horla (from the French *hors,* meaning "outside" and *de la,* meaning "there"), a being whom he comes to believe is at the vanguard of a group of extraterrestrials determined to subjugate humanity. The protagonist's journal entries reveal progressively more disturbing sensory experiences, while—to the reader—his sanity becomes increasingly suspect. Because of Maupassant's skill as a writer, it is not possible to know whether the encounter is merely a symptom of the protagonist's troubled mind or, conversely, whether his escalating anxiety is a natural consequence of the actual presence of the evil Horla (Lovecraft 1927).

This short story was published after some of the earliest reports of sleep paralysis appeared in the medical literature (e.g., Binns 1842; Mitchell 1876). The details of the encounter with the Horla are clearly consistent with descriptions of the traditional night-mare attack, but Maupassant's linking of sleep paralysis to psychological phenomena, such as anxiety and panic attacks, represents a shift away from earlier cultural understandings of the phenomenon.[1] "Le Horla" is an example of the way in which the increasing accessibility and popularization of scientific psychology in the nineteenth century provided new examples of and explanations for bizarre and uncanny experiences, including the nightmare (Cheyne n.d.).[2] In order to appreciate the pathopsychological trajectory of the night-mare over the past century, however, we must begin with the earliest psychoanalytic interpretations of the experience.

Pathologizing the Night-mare

When American writer Max Eastman visited Sigmund Freud's Vienna apartment in 1926, he noticed a print of John Henry Fuseli's *The Nightmare* hanging on the wall next to Rembrandt's *The Anatomy Lesson of Dr. Nicolaes Tulp* (Powell 1973)—"to express pictorially, perhaps, Freud's intention to render in medical terms what had always been seen as supernatural" (Thomas 1992, 70). Although Freud was surely aware of the night-mare, he does not directly address the phenomenon in his writings, focusing instead on dreams. In *The Interpretation of Dreams,* however, he does describe situations in which the sleeper feels that the ability to move is impaired:

> What is signified by the sensation of impeded movement, which so often occurs in the dream, and which is so closely allied to anxiety? One wants to move, and is unable to stir from the spot; or one wants to accomplish something, and meets one obstacle after another. . . . It is convenient, but inadequate, to answer that there is motor paralysis in sleep, which manifests itself by means of the sensation alluded to. . . . We are justified in supposing that this sensation, constantly appearing in sleep, serves some purpose or other in representation, and is brought about by a need occurring in the dream material for this sort of representation. . . . The sensation of impeded motion represents a *conflict of will.* (Freud 1903, 311–312)

Freud contends that, during such a dream, the sensation of inhibited motor movement represents the conflict between a desire for an action and the restraint of that action. After analyzing thousands of dreams, he became convinced that, without exception, "every dream represents the fulfillment in the imagination of some desire on the part of the patient, a desire that has either been 'repressed' in the waking state or else could not for some reason or other come to expression" (Jones 1931, 42). If the psychological conflict is so great that no compromise between the wish and its fulfillment can be reached, he reasons, then the sleeper awakens. Variations of this idea—the consequence of the sleeper's consciousness recognizing the nature of the repressed desire—would influence night-mare interpretation for decades.

In 1931, Ernest Jones, a member of Freud's inner circle and his official biographer, published his seminal work, *On the Nightmare.* Jones used psychoanalysis in an effort to bring new understanding to the phenomenon, which he believed to be central to human experience.[3] He was not satisfied with previous religious or physiological formulations of the disorder: "When clerical belief ascribed nightmares to evil spirits and medical to bodily disturbances they both absolved the subject's personality from any share in bringing them about" (1931, 7). Jones was particularly displeased with what he perceived to be inattention to the problem on the part of his medical colleagues:[4] "No malady that causes mortal distress to the sufferer, not even seasickness, is viewed by medical science with such complacent indifference as is the [night-mare]" (1931, 13).

Jones used the word *nightmare* in what he (correctly) considered to be its traditional sense: a phenomenon characterized by "(1) agonizing dread; (2) sense of oppression or weight at the chest . . . ; [and] (3) conviction of helpless paralysis" (Jones 1931, 52). Significantly, though, he did not include the impression of wakefulness as one of the defining characteristics of the night-mare. Because he did not recognize that the sensations occur in a semi-waking state, Jones characterized the context in which these symptoms are experienced as a type of disturbing dream. To be fair, Jones was writing before laboratory sleep research had revealed the stages of sleep, but the sharp distinctions between sleep paralysis and dreams could have been easily articulated by anyone who had experienced both. By not acknowledging the unique state of waking consciousness in which the night-mare occurs, Jones not only contributed to the long-standing scientific confusion over the significant differences between night-mares and "bad dreams" but also lost the opportunity to benefit from the firsthand knowledge of night-mare sufferers (Hufford 1982).

Jones began with the premise that night-mares are dreams; therefore, when his ideas were challenged by the traditional, historical descriptions of nightmare sufferers, he condescendingly concluded that "difficulty in distinguishing dreams from the experiences of waking life is naturally greater in less tutored minds, such as those of children and savages" (Jones 1931, 60).[5] Perhaps most importantly, however, by linking the concepts of night-mares and dreams, Jones's interpretations of the two became fused—bound together by Freud's theory of dreams and their meaning. To Jones, night-mare encounters were not simply rooted in the misunderstandings of the ignorant; they were signs of psychopathology.

Like Freud, Jones saw all dreams (including, erroneously, night-mares) as expressions of unconscious content, and he considered all fear represented in dreams to relate specifically to unconscious sexual conflicts.[6] Jones viewed the night-mare as a form of "*Angst* attack," due to an intense mental conflict regarding "a repressed component of the psycho-sexual instinct" (1931, 54).[7] As he wrote:

> Conflict of this fierce intensity never arises except over matters of sexuality, for on the one hand the sexual instinct is the source for most resistless desires and impulses, and on the other no feelings are repressed with such iron rigor as are certain of those that take their origin in this instinct. . . . The malady known as Nightmare is always an expression of intense mental conflict centering about some form of "repressed" sexual desire. . . . An attack of the Nightmare is an expression of the mental conflict over incestuous desire. (1931, 43–44)

To delineate the steps which comprise what appears to be a leap of logic: It was Jones's contention that, in the night-mare, dread reaches its maximum intensity. He believed that the source of the anxiety was located in the area of maximum repression or conflict. Jones insisted, moreover, that, in every case in which the night-mare had been psychoanalyzed, the difficulty could be traced to repressed incestuous desires, and that the introduction of this desire into consciousness was followed by the permanent cessation of the disorder.

Jones's approach represented a change from external spiritual and "physical explanations" for the night-mare to an emphasis on internal, psychological impairment: "In subjects who pass as being mentally normal, Nightmares never occur as isolated to morbid phenomena; on investigation it will always be found that other manifestations of *Angst* neurosis are present, with or without evidences of hysteria. In short, Nightmare may in such a subject be regarded as a symptom of this affection, and should be treated accordingly" (1931, 53). Following Jones, many investigators were interested in the influence that unconscious mental activity has on the subjective experience of night-mare symptoms. Subsequent researchers who studied the psychological significance of the nightmare conceptualized the phenomenon as an expression of mental conflict concerning areas as diverse as incestuous wishes, aggression, death, and sexual identity (Liddon 1970, 1030).[8]

Linking the Night-mare and Sleep Paralysis

The changing interpretations and understandings of the night-mare's features can be traced across different eras and in different cultural contexts. As we have seen, the night-mare has been ascribed to causes as diverse as demons and dyspepsia—and the attribution often reveals more about the sociopolitical environment than the actual phenomenon. The investigator's own understanding of the night-mare event not infrequently seems to function as a Rorschach inkblot test. Psychiatrist Jerome M. Schneck, in a 1948 article about the psychodynamics of sleep paralysis, discusses the case of a married, twenty-three-year-old man, who, notably, had no history of narcolepsy and presented with anxiety and a history of sleep paralysis. The patient, who had served overseas and been in combat for four months with an anti-aircraft unit, was a prisoner at a United States Disciplinary Barracks (for committing a robbery). Schneck describes the features of his case:

> The patient would doze, then find that he was unable to move; but he would groan and be awakened by others. The episodes probably lasted for a minute and a half to two minutes but to him the time seemed 15 minutes to an hour. On several occasions he had gone to sleep, keeping one foot near the edge of the bed, because, when the sleep paralysis set in, he might be able with great effort to force the foot off the bed, thus terminating the episode. When paralyzed, he would be aware that he was awake although unable to move, and he would be unable to open his eyelids. Bunk-mates at previous installations had been instructed by him simply to touch him when they heard him groan—in order to dispel the paralysis. (1948, 465)

The patient felt that he was awake, and knew where he was, but would experience auditory and visual hallucinations. On one occasion he heard

> someone come in through the barracks' door and walk the length of the floor toward his bed. He felt the bedcover being drawn from him and experienced the pressure of a knife against his chest. He could not identify the assailant, and his paralysis was complete. His groaning attracted attention, and he was assisted to awaken. At times the patient had had the hallucination that trucks were coming at him and that he was unable on his part to escape from their path. At other times, small airplanes dove directly at him. Once he felt he was walking along a trail. Japanese shot at him, hit him, and he could see the bullet holes. He attacked a Japanese and cut him. Other Japanese then attacked him with guns and bayonets. (Schneck 1948, 464–465)

Schneck explains that "consideration of the psychodynamics was stimulated by several facts pointing to the possible implication of latent homosexuality in symptom formation" (1948, 462–463).

> The hallucinatory episodes involving the trucks and airplanes, in themselves meaningless, may be allied to basic ambivalence toward homosexuality, with the panic that it instills, and the fear of assault. The episode of the Japanese attack, which may be connected with the war situation insofar as manifest elements are concerned, may nevertheless be associated likewise with mixed attitudes toward strong latent homosexual tendencies. The existence of associated anxiety could be substantiated by an interpretation of the symbolic significance of the assault by the person with a knife. The history of drinking in male company contributes affirmatively to the conjecture regarding the homosexual component. (Schneck 1948, 466)

This analysis is clearly (and quite ridiculously) tailored to a preconceived conclusion. It is much more likely that Schneck's examination simply exemplifies the misunderstandings that ensue when investigators unfamiliar with the night-mare's history, symptomatology, and epidemiology nevertheless attempt to interpret it.

Twentieth-century psychologists and psychiatrists have associated the night-mare with a variety of mental health and neurological concerns: neuroses, including personality conflicts characterized by indecision (Van Der Heide and Weinberg 1945), conflict between passivity and aggressivity (Payn 1965), and guilt about aggressivity (Levin 1961); psychoses (Liddon 1970); and even epilepsy (e.g., Ethelberg 1956; Rushton 1944). The majority of the anecdotal sleep paralysis cases reported in the medical literature from the 1940s to the 1960s, however, were interpreted as manifestations of a passive-aggressive conflict present in the patient's personality. In other words, during a sleep paralysis episode, the patient wants to move (be aggressive) but is unable to (remains passive) (e.g., Payn 1965; Schneck 1948; Van Der Heide and Weinberg 1945). Indeed, more than two decades after Schneck's first report on sleep paralysis, he himself noted that, although the initial data suggested the apparent importance of conflict over latent homosexuality, "subsequent studies strongly suggested the role of a broader issue involving conflict over opposing personality trends. Strivings toward active, aggressive functioning seemed to clash with leanings toward inactivity and passivity. The aggressivity-passivity problem is evidently expressed at certain times in the sleep paralysis attacks" (1957, 146).

Reports by other investigators soon confirmed that the occurrence of sleep paralysis (isolated from narcolepsy) was far more frequent than Schneck and other psychiatrists had realized. G. Browne Goode, for example, evaluated medical students, student nurses, and hospital in-patients and reported an incidence of

6.1 percent (1962). Henry C. Everett discovered that 15.4 percent of freshman medical students had had attacks of sleep paralysis (1963). This growing awareness that the frequency of the occurrence of sleep paralysis may have been underestimated provided a significant challenge to the exclusively psychopathological view of the night-mare.

A pivotal development in the understanding of the historical and cultural context of sleep paralysis came with the publication of Sim Liddon's "Sleep Paralysis and Hypnagogic Hallucinations: Their Relationship to the Nightmare" (1967). Liddon, an American psychiatrist, was one of the first to articulate the connection between the night-mare and sleep paralysis: "A full comparison of the present day reports . . . with the older descriptions of the nightmare, leaves little room to doubt that sleep paralysis and hypnagogic hallucinations were important features of the nightmare" (1967, 88). He notes that the night-mare and sleep paralysis "have other points of similarity besides the motor paralysis: severe anxiety is usually present in both conditions; . . . also, the feeling of suffocation so characteristic of the nightmare is at times described as accompanying sleep paralysis. But the most striking similarity is the fact that they both may be accompanied by a rather frightening hallucinatory experience" (1967, 89). Earlier researchers had conjectured that sleep paralysis may have "an organic substrate, which is used to express and solve emotional conflicts" (Payn 1965, 432), but Liddon goes a step further by suggesting that "the experience of sleep paralysis has no specific psychological meaning in itself and that it might be interpreted by different patients in different ways. . . . Such an idea would help explain the many different formulations about the psychological significance of sleep paralysis" (1970, 1031).

Liddon (like Jones before him) believed that sleep paralysis was associated historically with folk traditions, but it was not until the 1970s that researchers linked a culture-specific supernatural belief to sleep paralysis. It was David Hufford who published the first academic account of the congruence between the traditional pressing spirit of Newfoundland and sleep paralysis (1976); this was followed, two years later, by a corroborating article by sociologist Robert C. Ness (1978).[9] The work of these researchers in connecting traditional night-mares, as they were experienced by healthy people in the community, with episodes of sleep paralysis produced the data necessary to challenge earlier psychopathological assumptions.

As scientists became more aware of the night-mare's consistency across experiences (among different people) and how commonly it occurred in healthy individuals, the interpretation of night-mare attacks as signs of neurosis became more difficult to defend. First of all, it did not make sense that the consistent features of the night-mare experience among varied individuals were accounted for by a host of psychodynamic causes. Secondly, the night-mare experience simply seemed too prevalent to be characteristic of a disease process: "Any condition afflicting 15 percent or more of the general population, but remaining largely undiagnosed, must hopefully not be too serious" (Hufford 1982, 162). It began to appear more likely that researchers' lack of familiarity with the phenomenon's stability and frequency contributed to, if not created, the impression that the night-mare indicated the existence of pathology.[10]

The Night-mare and Current Issues in Mental Health

Even after researchers recognized the apparent universality of sleep paralysis, many psychologists and psychiatrists continued to emphasize that the obligatory neurophysiological features of sleep paralysis are used by individuals to express and solve mental conflicts (e.g., Payn 1965). We have seen that sleep paralysis can include auditory hallucinations (such as footsteps or verbal threats); visual hallucinations (an imposing, threatening figure); and sensations of pain, strangulation, extreme fear, and even impending death. The nature of these features has led some researchers to believe that the night-mare is implicated in contemporary psychological concerns. Two of these issues—memories of childhood sexual abuse and the experience of post-traumatic stress disorder—exemplify current psychological engagement with the night-mare.[11]

Memories of Childhood Sexual Abuse

Repressed memory is a theoretical concept that describes a significant memory—usually traumatic—that has become unavailable for recall. According to proponents of the theory, repressed memories may sometimes be recovered long after the event. The majority of these memories are spontaneously recovered in response to a variety of triggers, but they can apparently also be prompted through the use of memory recovering techniques, such as hypnosis and guided visualization. Critics of these methods, including mainstream psychologists and psychiatrists, are concerned that their use may result in patients "recalling" events that never occurred.

In *Victims of Memory: Sex Abuse Allegations and Shattered Lives,* investigative journalist Mark Pendergrast makes the highly controversial argument that some individuals who report recovered memories of childhood sexual abuse may have misinterpreted episodes of sleep paralysis as reemerging fragments of repressed memories (1996). In other words, some individuals may mistake sleep paralysis episodes for the nighttime resurfacing of dissociated fragments of buried memories of childhood sexual abuse. Pendergrast suggests that a person who experiences sleep paralysis that is accompanied by visions of a bedroom intruder and hallucinated bodily sensations might assume that he or she had been sexually victimized as a child, particularly in the absence of an alternative frame of reference. As one woman explained to him: "My eyes would just be open, and I would be frozen in terror in my bed, stiff. I couldn't even breathe. . . .

Well, I had never understood this, but now I connected it with the possibility of sexual abuse" (Pendergrast 1996, 259). In his book, Pendergrast reveals that he lost contact with his two adult daughters, apparently in connection with psychotherapy they received that involved repressed memories of childhood sexual abuse. Attempting to understand his own family's situation, Pendergrast noted a pattern of accusation and self-estrangement that follows unearthed "repressed memories of sexual abuse" in the United States and Canada. He argues that, in the late 1980s, people were encouraged by self-help books such as *The Courage to Heal* (Bass and Davis 1988), television talk shows, and therapists to believe that their problems as adults might stem from experiences of childhood sexual abuse.

Psychologist Ronald C. Johnson makes related claims in his examination of the psychological processes by which memories of satanic childhood sexual abuse were re-created in settings with counselors and ministers in the 1980s. Johnson asserts that satanic abuse allegations parallel alien abduction and historical witchcraft accusations in that the experiences are constructed into altered accounts by examiners' leading queries:

> The way repressed memories of childhood sexual abuse, including ritual satanic abuse, are restored and treated closely resembles the way memories are restored and treated in persons claiming to have been kidnapped by space aliens. The witchcraft trials in Salem have similarities to both of these. Persons claiming victimization learn of a possible cause for their distress and find specific persons to blame. They learn their symptoms from books, authority figures, or other "victims." Their beliefs are reinforced and validated by therapists, support groups, and, to varying degrees, the general community. (Johnson 1994, 41)

Johnson bases much of his analysis on Lawrence Wright's report, "Remembering Satan," in *The New Yorker* (Wright 1993). One of the memories recounted from this case is of a boy (Chad) who, as Johnson says, "eventually recalled being plagued by a witch, being bound and gagged" and sexually abused (Johnson 1994, 43). Chad's actual memory is of a repeated experience, detailed as follows:

> A witch would come in my window. . . . I would wake up, but I couldn't move. It was like the blankets were tucked under and . . . I couldn't move my arms. "You were being restrained?" Peterson [a psychologist] asked. Right, and there was somebody on top of me. . . . Chad then recalled that . . . he would find himself on the floor, and a fat witch with long black hair and a black robe would be sitting on top of him. (Wright 1995, 63)

The binding, gagging, and sexual abuse were inferences that the interrogators drew from what appears to be a recollection of a series of night-mare encounters.

Wright, interestingly, does not use the term *sleep paralysis* in his article; his only reference to the disorder is a brief mention of the Old Hag in a footnote (198).

It is concerning that when sexual abuse memories are recovered by therapists who are unfamiliar with the night-mare, a recollection of a sleep paralysis event can be interpreted as a "screen" that hides the real memory.

> These accounts share some striking consistencies because they are shaped by the sleep paralysis pattern that served as their starting point. I hasten to add that this observation does not in itself challenge the reality of either sexual abuse or even alien abduction. I have no doubt that the former occurs and no basis for a strong opinion about the latter. But it *does* challenge the use of clearly recognizable memories of sleep paralysis as in themselves either suggestive of abuse or abduction, or as a useful starting point for memory recovery. (Hufford 2005, 37)

Given the potential clinical, legal, and (above all) moral implications of associating sexual abuse with sleep paralysis, it is unfortunate that there is inadequate research on this subject. Psychologists Richard J. McNally and Susan A. Clancy conducted one of the few studies to examine the topic. A premise of their investigation was that an extremely distressing episode of sleep paralysis may be of sufficient intensity to elicit symptoms that could be mistaken as an emergent memory of an actual event. "Theoretically . . . sleep paralysis with its possible sexual connotations could result in false accusations of sexual abuse" (de Jong 2005, 90). McNally and Clancy's study was designed to explore Pendergrast's assertion; they asked four groups of adults who had previously participated in trauma and memory research to complete a questionnaire on sleep paralysis experiences. The participants included people who reported repressed, recovered, or continuous memories of childhood sexual abuse, in addition to a control group of individuals who had no reported history of childhood sexual abuse. "For those reporting childhood sexual abuse, episodes of sleep paralysis are generally negative experiences, in which people are left in a state of anger, sadness, and fear." Episodes of sleep paralysis are implicated by participants "as lingering after-effects of childhood sexual abuse, possibly as another form of reexperiencing. Whether episodes of sleep paralysis might be indicators of repressed childhood sexual abuse memories remains largely unexplored; however, negative sleep paralysis episodes do seem to be more prevalent among those who report childhood sexual abuse" (McNally and Clancy 2005, 600–601).[12] Clearly, as long as the night-mare remains largely unrecognized in a given cultural setting—either by the general public or by researchers—the controversy will continue.

Experiences of Post-traumatic Stress Disorder

Another psychological issue associated with the experience of sleep paralysis is post-traumatic stress disorder, a severe and ongoing emotional reaction to extreme trauma, such as being threatened with or experiencing great physical or psychological harm. Cambodian (Khmer) refugees have a high rate of post-traumatic stress disorder, as well as high rates of sleep paralysis. Devon Hinton, a psychiatrist and medical anthropologist at Harvard University, has conducted extensive research on sleep paralysis as a key dimension of the response to distress and trauma among Khmer refugee patients at a psychiatric clinic. The Cambodian term for sleep paralysis is *khmaoch sângkât,* "the ghost pushes you down": a dead person or supernatural being approaches the supine person and then puts a hand on the chest or neck, pushing down, causing chest tightness and making breathing difficult. Hinton presents several examples of *khmaoch sângkât,* including the case of Krauch, a forty-eight-year-old Khmer man who also experiences post-traumatic stress disorder:

> Krauch usually saw a black shape moving towards his body and, once it reached him, it seemed to wrap around him, severely impeding breathing. Krauch believed that the shape was either a demon or a ghost. In the week prior to his most recent clinic visit, Krauch had a new sleep paralysis visitor: a demon with fangs who held a nail-studded club. While Krauch was attempting to fall asleep, this new demon walked up to his side; he tried to move but couldn't. The demon pushed down on Krauch's chest with one hand, making him feel extremely short of breath. The demon then raised the club with the other hand, as if about to swing it down on Krauch's head; with its fangs protruding ominously close, the demon stood like this—one hand pushing down on Krauch's chest, the other holding the club above his head—for about two minutes. Then, just as the creature started to swing the club, Krauch was able to move. He sat up, seized by terror. For five minutes he felt his heart beat frantically, his ears rang, and his vision was blurry. . . . Krauch thought the being wanted to steal his soul by killing him directly or by scaring his soul out of his body. (Hinton et al. 2005, 54–55)

Hinton's research documents the highest rates of sleep paralysis reported in the literature: 60 percent of his Khmer patients with post-traumatic stress disorder experienced sleep paralysis (Hinton et al. 2009).[13] Hinton (as well as Bell, Dixie-Bell, and Thompson 1986; Ohayon et al. 1999; Paradis, Friedman, and Hatch 1997) suggests that panic disorder, post-traumatic stress disorder, and general stress greatly increase the rate of sleep paralysis. The very high prevalence of this parasomnia in the refugee Khmer population appears to be generated by cultural meanings and trauma resonances. Khmer believe that *khmaoch sângkât* is caused by various types of bodily dysfunction: "a dangerous weakness of the body; a 'weak heart' that may suddenly stop functioning properly, bringing about bodily 'freezing' (*keang*); an acute disturbance of the bodily flow of blood and a wind-like substance, or *khyâl*—*khyâl* runs alongside blood in vascular conduits—may cause a temporary (and quite possibly permanent) loss of limb function, as well as a dangerous surge of blood and *khyâl* upward in the body" (Hinton et al. 2005, 48).

During sleep paralysis, Khmer frequently see supernatural beings, such as a ghost sent by a sorcerer to kill the victim by putting objects into the body, a demon that wants to scare the soul from the body and cause death, or the ghost of someone killed during the Pol Pot regime. Hinton suggests that the figure seen in sleep paralysis may evoke trauma memories and survival guilt. The sensations experienced, particularly chest tightness and shortness of breath, may also recall "trauma memories encoded by the same sensations: near-drowning experiences; having a plastic bag placed over the head; being forced to carry heavy loads on the head or shoulders during the Pol Pot regime" (Hinton et al. 2005, 48).

Hinton's approach is instructive because, unlike earlier researchers of the psychopathology of the night-mare, he employs a method that respectfully engages the context of the patient's own understanding of the event. I have found that a willingness to use cross-cultural exploration (even in situations where the two "cultures" represented are simply those of health care professionals and patients) leads to awareness of the frequency of sleep paralysis, greater understanding of the distress sleep paralysis can cause, and the development of tailored interventions to ameliorate negative effects of sleep paralysis.

The Stigmatized Night-mare and Suppressed Reporting

The views that Ernest Jones expresses in *On the Nightmare* are typical of scholarly explanations that rely on the idea that people who experience night-mares are victims of both naïve thinking and psychopathology. Despite recent innovative research, these views remain common in some settings. It is a testament to the strength of cultural norms and expectations that such a widespread experience can remain hidden and misunderstood. When the night-mare is stigmatized, the reporting of encounters and sharing of experiences are suppressed. It seems likely that the majority of people in the United States who have had terrifying sleep paralysis experiences never told anyone about them—unless the individuals are part of a community that recognizes and can contextualize the attacks (such as groups with a strongly spiritual worldview).

When psychological aspects of the night-mare experience are investigated exclusively in people with mental health issues, researchers can draw the erroneous conclusion that the condition itself is a sign of psychopathology. Clearly, sleep paralysis may coexist with serious emotional disorders, but the tendency to look for study subjects among those previously diagnosed with psychopathology can reinforce a presumed connection. The mere co-occurrence of sleep paralysis and psychological problems does not prove causality. The psychoanalytic approach that considered sleep paralysis to be a sign of psychopathology (Payn 1965) has largely been abandoned (Kryger, Roth, and Dement 2000), but patients who do summon the courage to report a night-mare experience in a health-care setting still run the risk of having their accounts misinterpreted. These misunderstandings are not limited to American biomedical settings. Jude Uzoma Ohaeri, a psychiatrist at University College Hospital in Nigeria, describes the following case:

> This 37-year-old man is a top management executive of one of the multi-national companies and hails from a Muslim polygamous home of middle class status. He was referred by a neurologist. Since adolescence, he had been experiencing at least weekly attacks of isolated sleep paralysis. He had not worried about this because his father had similar problems, and in his father's case, the frequency of attacks reduced considerably with advancing years. But this man's own attacks were increasing in frequency with years. In his early undergraduate years in one of the local universities, he had been so worried by this problem that he had gone to sleep on the premises of one of the Pentecostal churches who had promised him "deliverance" from the spirits causing the isolated sleep paralysis. He stopped attending Christian faith healers because he had attacks of isolated sleep paralysis in all the nights he spent at the church. For many years thereafter, he continued to see only native doctors because the family opinion (which he agreed to) was that the problem was partly "spiritual," and they thought it would follow the same course as the father's. Eventually, the man had to see a doctor because he thought it was affecting his social functioning and a friend had suggested it might be "epilepsy." The isolated sleep paralysis experience alarmed him because in the midst of the paralysis, when he felt his life was most threatened, he could not even move his body to touch his wife sleeping beside him for help. This problem had so affected his life functioning that he was afraid of sleeping outside his home. On one occasion when he went to a conference at the new Federal capital of the north, he had to invite his driver to sleep with him in his five star hotel room. . . . Before being referred to the psychiatrist he had had a skull radiograph, two electroencephalograms, and biochemical investigations, all of which revealed no abnormality. (Ohaeri 1992, 522–523)

Ohaeri emphasizes that physicians "practicing in developing countries should take into consideration that fears of supernatural causation contribute to certain experiences in the clinical presentation of their patients" (522–523). Because these patients rarely spontaneously volunteer these fears, clinicians must develop the skill to elicit the information.

Night-mare sufferers who share their experiences anonymously as part of online sleep paralysis "communities" often describe situations in which they feel that physicians misattribute their night-mare symptoms. Concerns about these errors have been increasingly reported in the medical literature of the past decade. If the nature of sleep paralysis is not more widely understood, it seems likely that these diagnostic and treatment errors will continue to be made. Psychiatrists Sricharan Moturi and Anna Ivanenko note that "descriptions of hypnic hallucinations and sleep paralysis symptoms may lead to diagnostic misinterpretations of patients as psychotic, anxious, and/or depressed" (2009, 41), and they urge clinicians to "be aware that perceptual disturbances like hypnic hallucinations restricted to awakening and falling asleep are not sufficient to diagnose the patient with a psychotic disorder" (2009, 38). Researchers at the Medical University of South Carolina report findings from a case-control survey that indicate approximately 50 percent of psychiatrists (excluding those trained in sleep medicine) misdiagnosed sleep paralysis-related visual hallucinations as a "psychotic" disorder (Uhde, Merritt-Davis, and Yaroslavsky 2006). Night-mare sufferers' concerns appear to be well justified.

Internists, psychiatrists, and therapists approach their patients with a defined set of diagnostic categories—and night-mare or sleep paralysis are not typically among them. The problem of trying to fit diverse cultural experiences and interpretations into one nosological system is noted in the American Psychiatric Association's *Diagnostic and Statistical Manual of Mental Disorders:*

> A clinician who is unfamiliar with the nuances of an individual's cultural frame of reference may incorrectly judge as psychopathology those normal variations in behavior, belief, or experience that are particular to the individual's culture. For example, certain religious practices or beliefs (e.g., hearing or seeing a deceased relative during bereavement) may be misdiagnosed as manifestations of a Psychotic Disorder. (American Psychiatric Association 2000, xxxiv)

Significantly, sleep paralysis is no longer treated as a pathological condition, but as a parasomnia:

> Sleep paralysis: an inability to perform voluntary movement during the transition between wakefulness and sleep. The episodes may occur at sleep onset (hypnagogic) or with awakening (hypnopompic). The episodes are usually associated with extreme anxiety and, in some cases, fear of impending death. Sleep paralysis occurs commonly as an ancillary symptom of narcolepsy and, in such cases, should not be coded separately. . . . Most sleep-related hallucinations are visual and incorporate elements of the actual environment. For instance, individuals may describe objects appearing through cracks in the wall or describe objects moving in a picture on the wall. The hallucinations may also be auditory (e.g., hearing intruders in the home) or kinetic (e.g., sensation of flying) . . . Hypnagogic

and hypnopompic hallucinations are present in approximately 10–15 per-cent of the general population. . . . 40–50 percent of normal sleepers report having had isolated episodes of sleep paralysis at least once dur-ing their lifetime. Sleep-related hallucinations and sleep paralysis may occur simultaneously, resulting in an often terrifying experience of see-ing or hearing unusual things and being unable to move. (American Psychiatric Association 2000, 610)

This clear articulation of the non-psychopathological nature of sleep paralysis, together with the provision of a cross-cultural approach to psychiatric care, will hopefully increase sensitivity to the ways in which the night-mare may manifest in different cultural settings, as well as "reduce the possible effect of unintended bias stemming from the clinician's own cultural background" (American Psychiatric Association 2000, xxxiv).

In settings where there is no local tradition to legitimate sleep paralysis, the event may be interpreted by the experiencers themselves as evidence that they are—or are at risk of—becoming insane. When informed health-care providers use this opportunity to explain and provide a name for the sleep phenomenon, they find that their patients are (understandably) greatly relieved (Paradis, Friedman, and Hatch 1997). In the absence of a cultural framework, information alone may prove beneficial by helping individuals realize that sleep paralysis is experienced by a large percentage of the population (Wing, Lee, and Chen 1994).

4

The Night-mare in the Sleep Lab

"Besides waking life or sleeping life there is a third state, even more important for intercourse with the spiritual world. . . . I mean the state connected with the act of waking and the act of going to sleep, which last only briefly, for we immediately pass on into other conditions."

–Rudolf Steiner (1999, 152)

As a consequence of the laboratory sleep research of the mid-twentieth century, the night-mare was finally liberated from its exclusive association with psychiatric illness (Cheyne, Rueffer, and Newby-Clark 1999; Kryger, Roth, and Dement 2000). The first step in the de-pathologizing of the night-mare was the recognition of the ubiquity of sleep paralysis in the general population.[1] Most estimates of the prevalence of sleep paralysis are in the range of approximately 25 to 30 percent, but individual study findings vary considerably, with reports of 6 to 40 percent of healthy adults having experienced at least one episode of sleep paralysis (Arikawa et al. 1999; Awadalla et al. 2004; Buzzi and Cirignotta 2000; Cheyne, Newby-Clark, and Rueffer 1999; Cheyne, Rueffer, and Newby-Clark 1999; Fukuda et al. 1998; Kotorii et al. 2001; Ohayon et al. 1999; Spanos et al. 1995; Wing et al. 1999). It is not clear why there is such a wide range in reported rates, but some differences are likely due to the fact that many researchers make use of small, nonrandomized samples, as well as the fact that the wording of questions used to assess and categorize sleep paralysis is inconsistent across studies (Fukuda 1993; Ohayon et al. 1999). Perhaps most significantly, though, cultural context clearly contributes to the differences in reported prevalence. If a cultural category pertaining to sleep paralysis exists, it is more likely that the phenomenon will be reliably identified and reported to researchers. This is one reason that it is critical to balance the use of generic descriptions of sleep paralysis with the inclusion of local terms when conducting night-mare research. For example, psychologist Kazuhiko Fukuda and colleagues administered a sleep paralysis questionnaire to university students in Canada and Japan and found that, although there were no significant differences in the prevalence or symptoms of sleep paralysis, Canadian students tended to vaguely dismiss the experience as a "dream," whereas Japanese students clearly identified it as *kanashibari* (Fukuda et al. 1998).

The Sleep Ecology of Sleep Paralysis

Much of what is illuminating about considering scientific approaches to sleep paralysis is the comparison of purportedly "culture-free" experiences with instances of culturally embedded night-mares. A comparative strategy reveals key points of cultural variation not only in the night-mare, but also in the construct of sleep paralysis. Our current scientific understanding of sleep, for instance, is limited by the kinds of people that have been studied and by the contexts in which sleep has been investigated. Although all human beings sleep, not everyone sleeps in the same way. It has taken scientists an extraordinarily long time to realize that sleep is not purely "natural" (that is, biological) but is, in fact, deeply embedded in culture. Even anthropologists have only recently begun to consider the cultural context of sleep practices. How, when, and where do human beings sleep? Is sleep conducted in one sustained block of nocturnal time; in a biphasic manner, with a large period of nocturnal sleep and shorter afternoon one; or is it polyphasic, as in the so-called "napping cultures" of Japan and China? (Steger and Brunt 2003).

Sleep research has typically been conducted among middle-class Westerners who have grown up in and been habituated to a specific set of sleep ecologies.[2] These settings, although "successful research paradigms for elucidating dimensions of sleep patterning, physiology, regulation, and clinical correlates, may also of necessity and at times inadvertently eliminate variation that is crucial for understanding the full potential range of 'normal' sleep, as well as the causes and consequences of individual variability, normal and pathological" (Worthman and Melby 2002, 106). Distinctive features of these environments may influence the sleep behavior and physiology of research participants and thus affect both the resulting data and the models developed from them. Sleep laboratories, because of their aims as well as their locations, have provided a faithful reflection of the particular cultural ecology of Western sleep.

> Available sleep data generally are drawn from subjects who habitually sleep alone or with one other person and who have a developmental history of chronic solitary sleep. Western sleepers practice routinized bed- and wake-times strongly entrained to work or school, and again have done so throughout development. Hence, their sleep is highly bounded and consolidated, frequently restricted or curtailed by scheduling constraints, and preferably ungarnished by other forms of somnolence. Sleep is achieved and maintained in sensorily static and deprived (but potentially cognitively dense) conditions. In other words, the Western sleepers have lifetime habituation to many of the sleep conditions represented in the laboratory, and they tend to practice a "lie down and die" model of sleep. (Worthman and Melby 2002, 107)

The sleep patterns of most laboratory sleep subjects contrast sharply with those of people in many different parts of the world. In the United States, "patterns of solitary sleep on heavily cushioned substrates, consolidated in a single daily time block, and housed in roofed and solidly walled space" are quite distinct from the variety of sleep conditions found in many traditional societies, including "multiple and multi-age sleeping partners; frequent proximity of animals; embeddedness of sleep in ongoing social interaction; fluid bed times and wake times; use of the night time for ritual, sociality, and information exchange; and relatively exposed sleeping locations that require fire maintenance and sustained vigilance" (Worthman and Melby 2002, 70).

For the purposes of better understanding the night-mare, one of the most significant differences across cultural settings is the boundary between wakefulness and sleep. The distinction made between the two states is not uniform, and it seems to be linked to housing construction and patterns of social and ritual activity. "Sleep in . . . traditional societies is collective, and it occurs in social space; yet, at the same time, it is usually conventional to leave the sleeper alone, spared of undue disturbance, as the boundary of wake and sleep is fluid" (Worthman and Melby 2002, 79–80). The tradition of the wake/sleep dichotomy, of course, like that of the natural/supernatural world, is culturally and historically constructed and not universally accepted. The night-mare, by straddling what science teaches us are two distinct states—asleep and awake—violates our conception of consciousness. It is particularly disturbing because of the boundary that is so fiercely maintained between the rational (waking) and irrational or fanciful (sleep/dream). The scientific model of sleep status may thus represent a specific cultural approach that happens to highlight both ends of a spectrum and de-emphasize the intervening gradations. "In other societies, sleep behaviorally, and perhaps conceptually, may be on a continuum of arousal where other modes (from, for instance, disengaged semialert, to somnolence or drowsing, to dozing, to napping) are more tolerated and perhaps more prevalent" (Worthman and Melby 2002, 102). This cross-cultural diversity in sleep patterns and ecologies is significant because specific cultural settings and practices may be associated with distinctive risks for disorders of sleep.

Sleep Paralysis as a Biologically Structured Event

The (Re)Discovery of the REM Sleep Period

Perhaps the single most important event for the biomedical understanding of the night-mare was the discovery of the periodically occurring rapid eye movement (REM) sleep phase. Although it was commonly understood that eye movements often accompany sleep, no one had recorded eye movements throughout the course of an entire night's sleep. In 1953, after spending countless hours observing sleeping infants as part of his graduate work, Eugene Aserinsky applied polygraph technology to the study of nocturnal eye movements. In his early experiments, Aserinsky enlisted the aid of his own eight-year-old son. What he discovered was so unexpected, that for some time he suspected that the equipment was malfunctioning. "I noticed to my chagrin that the machine was acting up again, [with some recordings] that looked suspiciously like the saccades I had observed when my son moved his eyes voluntarily during the calibration prior to sleep" (Aserinsky 1996, 217). Because of this seemingly anomalous finding, Aserinsky was compelled to reconsider a limited number of possibilities for the cause of these eye movements, including what he considered the least likely, that the "hoary anecdotal reports tying eye movements to dreaming might indeed be true" (217).[3] Aserinsky recalls from his subsequent work with sleeping adults: "In one of the earliest sleep sessions, I went into the sleep chamber and directly observed the eyes through the lids at the time that the sporadic eye movement deflections appeared on the polygraph record. The eyes were moving vigorously, but the subject did not respond to my vocalization. There was no doubt whatsoever that the subject was asleep despite the EEG [electroencephalogram] suggesting a waking state" (218).[4]

Stages of Sleep

As a result of the foundational sleep studies conducted in the mid-1950s, sleep researchers began to differentiate between two categories of sleep, Rapid Eye Movement (REM) and Non-Rapid Eye Movement (NREM), each with what are now recognized as a characteristic set of physiological, neurological, and psychological features. REM sleep is distinguished by brain waves resembling those of wakefulness. In contradistinction to the waking state, however, the body is paralyzed, apparently to keep the sleeper from acting out his or her dreams.[5] Sleep typically is arranged in ninety-minute cycles consisting of three stages of progressively deeper NREM sleep, followed by one stage of REM. (A system for staging sleep was established in 1968 by Allan Rechtschaffen and Anthony Kale, and it remained officially unchanged until the American Academy of Sleep Medicine updated the staging guidelines [Iber, Ancoli-Israel, Chesson, et al. 2007].)

Stage N1 (for NREM 1) sleep is a phase of somnolence or drowsiness. Polysomnography shows a 50 percent reduction in activity between wakefulness and this first stage of sleep. The eyes are closed and the "sleeper" loses some muscle tone and conscious awareness of the external environment, but, if aroused from N1, a person may feel as if he or she has not slept. Stage N1 lasts for five to ten minutes. Sudden twitches and muscle jerks (known as positive myoclonus) are also associated with the onset of sleep during N1. The muscles begin to slack and go into a restful state as a person is falling asleep. The brain apparently senses these relaxation signals and misinterprets them, thinking the sleeper is falling down. The brain then sends signals to the muscles in the arms and legs in an attempt to jerk the body back upright.[6] Psychologist Frederick Coolidge suggests that this is a vestige from our time as tree-dwelling primates, when there was a selective value to readjusting sleeping positions to prevent a fall (Coolidge 2006).[7]

Stage N2 is a period of light sleep during which muscular activity decreases, heart rate slows, body temperature decreases, and conscious awareness of the external environment disappears. At this point, the body prepares to enter deep sleep. N2 comprises 45–55 percent of total sleep.

Stage N3/4 is characterized by deep and slow-wave sleep. Night terrors, bed-wetting, sleepwalking, and sleep-talking occur during this phase. Stage N4 had previously been thought of as a deeper version of N3, in which the deep-sleep characteristics are more pronounced. Under the new AASM guidelines, how-ever, the distinction between Stages 3 and 4 of NREM sleep is viewed as incon-sequential and both are considered slow-wave sleep. As of 2007, therefore (in an effort to increase the precision of sleep scoring guidelines), stage N4 is no longer officially coded separately in AASM sleep centers.

REM sleep is easily distinguished from NREM sleep by physiological changes, including the characteristic rapid eye movements. Polysomnograms, however, show brain-wave patterns in REM to be similar to those of NI sleep. In normal sleep (that is, in people without disruptions of sleep-wake patterns or REM behavior disorder), a person's heart and respiration rates accelerate and become erratic, while his or her face, fingers, and legs may twitch. Because of heightened brain activity, intense dreaming occurs during REM sleep, but paralysis occurs simultaneously in the major voluntary muscle groups. Since REM sleep is thus a combination of states of brain excitement and muscular immobility, it is some-times called "paradoxical sleep" (Jouvet 2001). REM-associated muscle paralysis (or atonia) functions to prevent the body from acting out the dreams that occur during this intensely cerebral stage. In a typical night's sleep, the first period of REM lasts ten minutes, and each recurring REM phase lengthens until the final one lasts one hour. REM sleep is also homeostatically driven—if a person is deprived of sleep, there are progressively more frequent attempts to enter REM and a compensatory rebound after the sleep deprivation ends.

How the Night-mare Manifests in the Sleep Lab

Sleep paralysis may occur during sleep-onset or sleep-offset REM (Hishikawa and Shimizu 1995), the result of a REM state that occurs "out of sequence" while the sleeper is still partially conscious. This overlap causes sleep paralysis, a stage in which the body is asleep but the mind is not. The best way to understand this state is to think of REM characteristics, including muscle atonia, overlaid on wak-ing consciousness. (See Illustration 4.1 for a depiction of a "sleeper" paralyzed during a night-mare.) Often, sleep paralysis is also accompanied by dream-like hallucinations which consist of complex visual, auditory, and somatosensory per-ceptions that occur as a person is falling asleep (in which case the hallucinations are referred to as hypnagogic, from the Greek words *hypnos* ["sleep"] and *agogos*

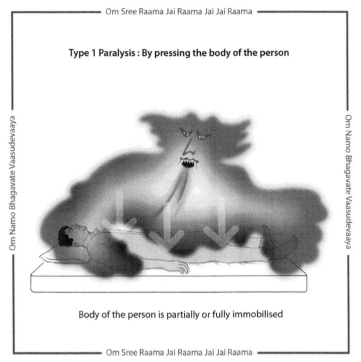

Om Sree Raama Jai Raama Jai Jai Raama

Type 1 Paralysis : By pressing the body of the person

Om Namo Bhagavate Vaasudevaaya

Om Namo Bhagavate Vaasudevaaya

Body of the person is partially or fully immobilised

Om Sree Raama Jai Raama Jai Jai Raama

4.1. Depiction of Immobilization during Sleep Paralysis. This illustration was provided by the Spiritual Science Research Foundation (SSRF), a nonprofit organization that, over the past twenty years, has conducted spiritual research. A representative of SSRF explained that the organization's intention is "to demystify the spiritual realm and provide research that will help humanity to effectively alleviate difficulties in life and progress spiritually in a very practical manner." The text circumscribing the illustration is a Sanskrit mantra. The chants are "a subtle protective border which does not allow negative energies to spread their black energy onto anyone who is looking at the drawing. The visual drawing of a negative energy also carries its associated energy. So we kindly suggest that those chants remain."

© Spiritual Science Research Foundation, www.ssrf.org.

["leading"]) or waking up (hypnopompic hallucinations, from *pompe* ["procession"]). Both David Hufford (1976, 1982) and Robert Ness (1978) argue convincingly that these out-of-place REM stages account for the subjective impression of wakefulness, the feeling of paralysis, and, understandably, the tremendous anxiety that mark the night-mare experience. It is important to remember that paralysis is a normal physiological correlate of REM sleep; it is the consciousness of the paralysis that is "abnormal."

More recent research has confirmed and elaborated upon earlier findings regarding the relationship between night-mare encounters and sleep-onset/ offset REM. For example, features of the night-mare are consistent with several

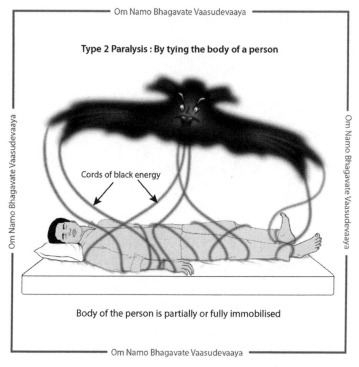

4.2. Depiction of Pressure during Sleep Paralysis.

© Spiritual Science Research Foundation, www.ssrf.org.

characteristics of REM respiration, including shallow rapid breathing, hypoxia (an inadequate oxygen supply), hypercapnia (a high level of carbon dioxide in the blood), and occlusion of the airways (Cheyne, Rueffer, and Newby-Clark 1999). Both tidal volume and breathing rate are sometimes quite variable during REM sleep, and because major anti-gravity muscles are paralyzed, the chest contributes less to breathing during REM than during NREM sleep (Douglas and Polo 1994). Even in the absence of apnea or blood chemistry changes, people will sometimes attempt to breathe deeply, just as they try to make other movements during sleep paralysis (Hishikawa and Shimizu 1995). When a sleeper's efforts to control breathing are unsuccessful, the sense of resistance can be interpreted as pressure. (Illustration 4.2 depicts the "pressure" of a night-mare attack.) The sense of oppression or weight on the chest and the common feature of lying in a supine position can be explained by the fact that when the sleeper is on his or her back, the atonic muscles of the tongue and esophagus collapse the airway. The relaxed muscles not only hinder breathing, but they can also create a sensation of pressure or strangulation (Adler 1994). The awareness of increased airflow resistance that can occur during sleep paralysis leads to panic and strenuous efforts to regain control (Cheyne, Rueffer, and Newby-Clark 1999).

In addition to these common night-mare features that fit into the known neurophysiology of REM sleep, the sexual nature of some night-mare encounters may be similarly related to REM characteristics. If physiological processes are elaborated into night-mare content generally, then the same is likely true for the concomitant occurrence of increased sexual arousal in women and men during the REM stage. The occurrence of sexual processes in sleep-onset/offset REM may thus be incorporated by the semiconscious mind into the experience of the night-mare.

During sleep paralysis, individuals are aware of their surroundings and can open their eyes, but they are unable to move (Hishikawa 1976). Not surprisingly, an acute sense of fear or doom often accompanies the various hypnagogic and hypnopompic experiences that occur with sleep paralysis. For the sake of simplicity, I will use the term *hypnic* to indicate the timing of these strange sensory experiences, whether they occur upon falling asleep or awakening. Sleep paralysis hallucinations are, in effect, the "superpositioning of dream imagery and affect on waking consciousness" (Cheyne 2001, 134). These hypnic experiences include a strong sense of a monitoring "evil presence"; combinations of auditory and visual hallucinations; pressure on the chest; and sensations of suffocating, choking, floating, flying, and being "out of body" (Hishikawa 1976; Hufford 1976). Although these features are in some ways similar to images and sensations that are unrelated to sleep paralysis (e.g., Foulkes and Vogel 1965; Mavromatis 1987; Rowley, Stickgold, and Hobson 1988; Schacter 1976), hypnic experiences that occur with sleep paralysis seem to be significantly more intense and horrifying (Cheyne, Newby-Clark, and Rueffer 1999; Hufford 1982; Takeuchi et al. 1992). In spite of the compelling nature of hypnic hallucinations, however, people may be easily aroused from the state of sleep paralysis by external tactile and auditory input (Hishikawa 1976)—typically a touch by someone who has noticed the sleeper's distress.

What the Night-mare Is Not: Night Terrors, Bad Dreams, and Narcolepsy

The problem of distinguishing the night-mare experience from other sleep disorders—particularly night terrors, bad dreams, and narcolepsy—persists. Ironically, "folk observation is ahead of scientific observation. Without sleep laboratories and without polygraphs, folk tradition apparently maintained an awareness of the distinction between REM intrusions into wakefulness and REM occurring in its proper places" (Hufford 1982, 166). The night-mare experiencers' observations were correct; they were "awake," and they were having anomalous experiences. Scholars' rejection of this observation delayed progress in night-mare research and resulted in much scientific confusion.

Even the most preposterous explanation should not prevent us from seriously considering an observation repeatedly made by large numbers of our fellow humans, whatever their education. It was just such a rejection of untutored observation that delayed for so long the "scientific" discovery of giant squid, gorillas, meteors, and any number of other wild and wonderful (but apparently unlikely) facts of this world. In those cases, *post hoc* scientific rationalization was used to explain how people came to believe in such things. Seasoned fishermen were said to mistake floating trees with large root systems for huge animals attacking their boats; farmers were said to have overlooked large iron-bearing rocks in the midst of their fields until they were pointed out by lightning; and in this case, "children and savages" were said to have difficulty knowing when they were awake and when they were asleep. (Hufford 1982, 166)

Given the continuing confusion, further misunderstandings are probably best prevented by considering recent findings in sleep research in order to differentiate among the three parasomnias, or sleep disorders, most often confused with the night-mare: night terrors, bad dreams, and narcolepsy. Sleep paralysis, as we have seen, is the result of REM atypically intruding into N1 sleep. Night terrors or sleep terrors, in contrast, are spontaneous awakenings from N3/4 sleep, usually during the first one-third of the sleep period. Night terrors, which occur most frequently in childhood, manifest when a person sits up in bed with a loud scream or cry and a look of intense fear. Adults may jump out of bed and run, attempting to leave through a door or window. The "sleeper" is typically unresponsive and will be confused and disoriented if awakened. Any efforts to console the person only prolong or intensify the episode. There is usually no memory of the incident in the morning. About 2 percent of adults and up to 6 percent of children experience night terrors (Schenck 2007).

Generic bad dreams (or, confusingly, "nightmares" in everyday language) are disturbing mental experiences that occur during REM and often result in awakenings from sleep. Bad dreams have coherent narrative sequences that seem real and become increasingly more disturbing as they unfold. These dreams tend to focus on imminent physical danger or other distressing themes. Anxiety or fear is typically associated with these experiences, but emotions of anger, rage, embarrassment, and disgust are common. In addition, the fear that is provoked by a bad dream is qualitatively different than the intense horror and sense of doom that are common results of the night-mare encounter. The sleeper is often able to recall clear details of a bad dream after awakening, and there is little confusion or disorientation (Schenck 2007).

Unlike the other parasomnias, narcolepsy is associated with sleep paralysis in some individuals, but isolated sleep paralysis is overwhelmingly more prevalent in the general population. Narcolepsy is a neurological sleep disorder that creates a potentially disabling level of daytime sleepiness. The cause of most cases of narcolepsy is the loss of neurons that contain hypocretin, a protein that helps the brain maintain alertness (Schenck 2007). This sleepiness may take the form of repeated and irresistible bouts of sleep, during which a person suddenly falls asleep in unusual situations, such as while eating, walking, or driving. Most people tested with narcolepsy fall asleep in an average of less than eight minutes (often less than five minutes). They also show a tendency to enter the REM stage of sleep much faster than normal sleepers—it is this feature that results in narcoleptics' relatively high rate of sleep paralysis. The primary distinguishing features of most cases of narcolepsy are excessive daytime sleepiness (inability to stay awake and alert during the major waking periods of the day), cataplexy (a sudden loss of muscle tone that occurs most often in the knees, face, and neck), sleep paralysis, and hypnagogic hallucinations (Kryger, Roth, and Dement 2000). Less than 1 percent of the general population has narcolepsy, compared with 25–30 percent who experience sleep paralysis.

Sleep Paralysis and the Night-mare

Sleep paralysis and the night-mare are the same phenomenon described and experienced through different paradigms (biomedical versus cultural). Some of the most innovative and important work in reconciling the neurophysiology of sleep paralysis with the experience of the night-mare has been conducted by psychologist J. Allan Cheyne and his colleagues at the University of Waterloo in Ontario. In order to study what Cheyne refers to as "waking nightmares" in the general population, he developed the Waterloo Unusual Sleep Experiences Questionnaire, which has been completed by over 12,000 respondents to date. The primary purpose of the survey is to assess the frequency and intensity of sleep paralysis, as well as the qualitative features of the hallucinatory experiences that frequently accompany sleep paralysis. The questionnaire assesses respondents' experience with a range of hypnic occurrences, including sensed presence; visual and auditory hallucinations; pressure on the chest; difficulty breathing; pain, choking, or smothering; motor movements (e.g., getting up, walking around, flipping light switches); floating, out-of-body experiences, falling, "elevator feelings," flying, or spinning sensations; and autoscopy (observing one's body from a perspective outside of the physical self). The questionnaire also assesses fear, anger, sadness, bliss, and erotic feelings. Respondents are asked to rate the intensity and frequency of each type of experience.

Cheyne and his research team found a high degree of structure in the patterning of hypnic experiences, with a clustering into three primary groups: (1) sensed presence, fear, and auditory and visual hallucinations; (2) pressure on the chest, breathing difficulties, and pain; and (3) "unusual bodily experiences," consisting of floating/flying sensations, out-of-body experiences, and feelings of bliss. A sensed presence is the most common experience reported, and fear is the most frequently noted emotion. The researchers emphasize that many respondents spontaneously reported that they had never spoken to anyone about their experiences because they were afraid that they might be considered "weird." The survey participants "also indicated that they had thought their experiences were unique and expressed considerable relief upon discovering this was a known phenomenon" (Cheyne, Newby-Clark, and Rueffer 1999, 316).

Sleep research offers a scientific explanation for the major features of the night-mare and it accounts for other common elements, such as the "evil presence." We know that the motor paralysis of REM can lead to the experience of breathing difficulties when a sleeper tries to inhale deeply, and that this is sometimes experienced as sensations of choking or suffocating. This inability to breathe deeply may also be interpreted by the sleeping brain as being caused by a weight or pressure on the chest. From a sleep science perspective, there is a cascading series of events initiated by motor inhibition that lead to experiences of breathing difficulties, pressure on the chest, and ultimately a sense of physical assault (Cheyne, Rueffer, and Newby-Clark 1999). The impression of a nearby threatening presence with corroborating visual and auditory evidence provides an "agent" to perpetrate the experienced assault: "The mapping is such that little needs to be added to this cluster of [sleep-onset/offset REM] experiences and everything available fits well with a narrative of assault by a strange intruder" (Cheyne, Rueffer, and Newby-Clark 1999, 333).

Cheyne and colleagues propose that the major initiating event of hallucinations of a nearby, threatening person or entity is the experience of a sensed presence accompanied by intense fear. As the sleep paralysis episode continues, the sensed presence provokes continuing efforts to establish the true meaning of the experience, as well as increasingly elaborate interpretations of accompanying hypnic hallucinations consistent with an external threat. In other words, the brain strives desperately to make meaning out of the anomalous sensations. The hallucinations can arise from within the body, through ocular or middle ear activity, or from outside the body as shadows and ambient sounds. These sensations are frequently interpreted as "approaching footsteps, whispering voices, or apparitions that are taken to be concrete instantiations of the threatening presence" (Cheyne, Rueffer, and Newby-Clark 1999, 322).

In contrast to experiences centered on an evil presence or sense of pressure, other hypnic sensations do not necessarily imply threatening external agency but are instead associated with bodily orientation and movement in space. These experiences are typically not passive sensations; they consist of more vigorous sensations of flying, acceleration, and "even wrenching of the 'person' from his or her body." In response to questions about these sensations, study participants "spontaneously reported a variety of inertial forces acting on them, which they described as rising, lifting, falling, flying, spinning, and swirling sensations or similar to going up or down in an elevator or an escalator, being hurled through a tunnel, or simply accelerating and decelerating rapidly" (Cheyne, Rueffer, and Newby-Clark 1999, 331).

In the waking state, the vestibular system is responsible for our balance and sense of spatial orientation. During REM, activity in the vestibular system increases, but, because the body is asleep, this activity occurs in the absence of accurate information about the position and motion of the body and limbs. In other words, the natural vestibular activation of REM occurs without corroborating somatosensory information or with conflicting information. In the absence of (accurate) feedback, the resulting sensations are interpreted as floating or flying or one of a number of other unusual bodily sensations (Cheyne and Girard 2008). This irreconcilable conflict between moving and not moving "is resolved by a splitting of the phenomenal self and the physical body, sometimes referred to as an out-of-body experience" (Cheyne, Rueffer, and Newby-Clark 1999, 331). (One does not have to be in an anomalous state for the vestibular system to become confused. If you are sitting in a train at rest in a station when the train on the next track begins to move, the conflicting sensory input is likely to cause you to experience a vivid, if brief, illusion of movement.)

Although out-of-body experiences, especially those accompanying trauma and/or seizures, can be associated with fear (Devinsky et al. 1989), studies in broader populations find that some people describe feelings of calm, peace, and joy that are sufficiently positive to create the desire to repeat these experiences. This positive association seems to be particularly common among people who practice meditation and find themselves able to experience a feeling of transcendence (Cheyne 2001).

The Primordial Narrative of the Threatening Intruder

Cheyne and colleagues present the intriguing hypothesis that the sensed presence and related hallucinations in the sleep paralysis arise from hypervigilant defensive states initiated in the mid-brain. Under these circumstances, the sleeper is extraordinarily alert to environmental events potentially associated with danger. The feelings of presence that emerge during sleep paralysis thus arise from the same neurophysiology that underlies threat detection.

> The sensed presence is typically described as a monitoring one, akin to a predator stalking its prey. A threatening, malignant or evil intent is frequently ascribed to the presence. Respondents are often at pains to express the intensity and depth of the accompanying terror. In addition, bodily sensations of crushing and painful pressure on the chest, back, side and neck may be interpreted as a full-fledged and potentially mortal attack by the presence. (Cheyne, Rueffer, and Newby-Clark 1999, 322)

During sleep paralysis, REM-based activation of the vigilance system produces (in the absence of an external threat) an ambiguity that cannot be conventionally resolved—this condition is experienced as an extremely threatening sensed presence. During sleep-onset/offset REM, the sensed presence may serve to give meaning to the visual and auditory hallucinations that are occurring simultaneously. When the "triggers" are internal, the sense of threat cannot be immediately corroborated and the sleeper's sense of fear takes on an otherworldly quality and intensity. I would suggest, in addition, that as the brain frantically attempts to comprehend why its motor commands are not being followed, a spiral of increasingly fearful thoughts is formed. This is, in essence, a type of nocebo effect: through the "power of negative thinking," the vague sense of threat and its anticipated horror are realized.

Visual hallucinations thus may represent attempts by the brain's threat detection mechanisms to explain and literally "flesh out" the sensed presence. Auditory hallucinations (e.g., approaching footsteps, demonic whispering) may similarly arise from the results of random activation of auditory centers during REM that are made "meaningful" by the brain. It is clear from talking with night-mare sufferers, though, that even when the hallucinations provide an "explanation" of the event, it is, at best, only an incomplete resolution of the anomaly—and the night-mare experience retains its otherworldly quality. It is very common for night-mare sufferers to spontaneously and strenuously assert that the terror they experience is unlike any real-world fear that they have ever known. This terror is evocative of the "numinous" sensation described by the theologian and religious scholar Rudolf Otto as the ineffable sense of a sacred or demonic presence (1926). Otto explains that a sensed encounter with the supernatural causes a numinous reaction that is qualitatively different from all other emotions. The combination of fear, awe, and abasement in the presence of a greater power (such as that which a person feels during a supernatural encounter) forms a composite emotion that is like no other (Adler 1991). The experience of the numinous is one of "terror fraught with an inward shuddering such as not even the most menacing and overpowering created thing can instill" (Otto 1926, 14).

Stress and Sleep Disruption as Precursors to Sleep Paralysis

Findings from sleep research offer explanations not only for the features of the night-mare, but also for its causes and "cures." Stress, anxiety, sleep disturbances, and sleep deprivation (which often co-occur) are the most common precursors of sleep paralysis.[8] When interviewed about the night-mare, people often spontaneously mention that they were under a lot of stress during episodes. Periods of stress are associated with difficulty falling asleep (leading to sleep deprivation), as well as multiple and extended awakenings during the night and early waking (both of which have a relatively greater impact on REM sleep). Insufficient amounts of REM sleep can lead to sleep onset-REM in subsequent sleep. People who do shift work or night work have been shown to suffer from disrupted sleep-wake patterns, sleep deprivation, and, not surprisingly, sleep paralysis (Kotorii et al. 2001). The situation is sufficiently common among nurses who work long and irregular shifts that it has been known as "night nurse paralysis" (Folkard, Condon, and Herbert 1984). Nurses have reported becoming aware of these sleep paralysis episodes when a patient calls and they find themselves unable to move to respond to the request. There are many other work-related situations in which there are enormous safety implications for people who find themselves incapacitated by sleep paralysis, including those of air traffic controllers (Folkard and Condon 1987)[9] and physicians (Weinger and Ancoli-Israel 2002).

The historical record seems to confirm that stress, anxiety, and strenuous activity—because they involve irregular sleep—increase the chances of sleep paralysis. There is an account of a panic in Breslau (modern-day Wrocław, Poland) during the late sixteenth century that was caused by visitations of the ghost of a shoemaker who had committed suicide. The revenant came to some people at night, lay on them, and smothered and "squeezed" them hard. The people "most bothered were those who wanted to rest after heavy work" (Barber 1988, 12). In another example, during the late nineteenth century, an elderly Scottish woman explained: "When the females of a house had all the work, and were 'stinted' to do a given amount of work at the spinning wheel before they got any supper, and so much before they went to bed, they were very liable to take the 'Mare' owing to anxiety connected with their stints" (Ducie 1888, 135).[10] Even today, accounts of night-mare experiences often include a description of irregular sleep. According to one American soldier: "Being in the army, my sleep patterns are very 'scattered.' I usually get 4 hours a night at different times and I nap during the day whenever I can. I get sleep paralysis on average once to twice a week. I HATE IT. You don't want this to happen to you. It scares the daylights out of me every time I experience it. I feel like I'm dead" (Internet posting, ASP-L).

The impact of age is another factor in the occurrence of sleep paralysis. Tsuyoshi Kotorii and colleagues conducted a sleep survey with more than eight thousand people in Japan and found that "many young people have irregular life rhythms or delayed sleep, and there is the possibility that disturbances in sleeping and awakening rhythm may increase the experience rate of sleep paralysis. . . . Although the frequency of insomnia increases with age, the cumulative experience rate of sleep paralysis decreases with age" (Kotorii et al. 2001, 266).[11] The greater the degree of insomnia, the higher the cumulative experience rate of sleep paralysis. The interruption of sleep caused by insomnia and higher levels of anxiety appear to increase the cumulative experience rate of sleep paralysis.

There have been a host of reports in both the scientific and popular media in recent years that call attention to the prevalence and dangers of chronic sleep deprivation (e.g., Revill 2006; Van Dongen et al. 2003). Any kind of stress can be disruptive of sleep patterns, but when the stressor itself is the interruption of sleep, the effect is significantly more dramatic. Repeated episodes of sleep deprivation/disruption and sleep paralysis may create a vicious cycle. It is ironic that life in the contemporary United States removes many cultural narratives that give meaning to the events of sleep paralysis but creates conditions that increase its incidence.[12]

Preventing Sleep Paralysis

In the absence of cultural traditions, the Internet is a resource for popular suggestions about how to elude sleep paralysis. One British Web site makes the following representative recommendations: "Keep to a regular schedule. Go to bed and get up at regular times. Eat your meals at regular times. Get some exercise, although not too close to bedtime. Avoid sleep deprivation—make sure you get enough sleep. Find ways to reduce stress in your life. Try to avoid sleeping on your back" (Sleep Paralysis Information Service 2009). With the exception of avoiding the supine position, suggestions like these are indistinguishable from contemporary generic tips for "healthy living," and they have not progressed far from the advice commonly given more than two centuries ago:

> If the disorder proceed from heavy suppers, or indigestible food, these things ought to be given up, and the person should either go supperless to bed, or with such a light meal as will not hurt his digestion. . . . In all cases, the patient should take abundant exercise, shun late hours . . . and keep his mind in as cheerful a state as possible. . . . He should be directed to lie as little as possible on the back. (MacNish 1834, 27)

Strategies suggested by contemporary sleep scientists for preventing sleep paralysis also overlap with traditional actions taken against the night-mare. Since lying in a supine position is five times more likely during sleep paralysis than during normal sleep, people hoping to prevent the disorder are advised to avoid sleeping on their backs. Sleeping supine, however, appears to be relatively rare—for example, only 10–15 percent of people in a large Canadian study reported that they normally sleep in this position (Cheyne 2002). Because about 60 percent of sleep paralysis episodes are reported to occur in the supine position, many people clearly find themselves in what is for them an atypical sleep position.[13] Unfortunately, this means that people who experience sleep paralysis may be no more likely to be lying on their backs when normally falling asleep than people who do not experience them. (In addition, those who typically fall asleep on their backs do not report greater frequency of sleep paralysis or associated hallucinations.) Sleep paralysis thus usually occurs when susceptible individuals inadvertently turn to the supine position as they fall asleep or when they change positions during sleep, particularly when they enter or leave the REM stage. Avoiding the supine position only when falling asleep, therefore, is not enough. To address this problem, scientists and clinicians sometimes recommend the "sleep-ball" or "tennis-ball technique," which originated as a remedy for positional sleep apnea (Skinner et al. 2008). In this technique, a tennis ball is placed in a pocket that has been sewn onto the back of pajamas or placed in a sock that is safety-pinned to the back of a nightshirt, thus preventing the night-mare sufferer from sleeping comfortably on his or her back.

In addition to altering sleep position, another preventive measure based on sleep research, but familiar from folk tradition, is the attempt to make small motions to end the episode. As psychiatrist Carlos Schenck describes: "Your bigger muscles may be frozen, but it may be possible to direct the smaller ones—the fingers and toes in particular. Often just one small movement of a finger is enough to break the paralysis. If you can't move your fingers, try shifting the eyes back and forth" (Schenck 2007, 174). Finally, the centuries-old strategy of avoiding overindulgence in food or drink before bed is still strongly advised (Cheyne 2002).

Luring the Night-mare: Inducing Sleep Paralysis

Every aspect of sleep paralysis does not necessarily map onto each night-mare experience. The range of sleep paralysis symptoms is broader than the defining features of a night-mare—and the feeling of weight or pressure that is often a central feature of the night-mare encounter is not always a component of sleep paralysis experiences. People describe a number of different sensations during the transition to or from sleep, including flying, rising, spinning, accelerating, and hurtling through a tunnel—all sensations that, although not part of a classic night-mare encounter, may (albeit rarely) accompany sleep paralysis. An even smaller proportion of people describe out-of-body experiences in which they float above their beds and look down on their own bodies. Remarkably, this experience is usually described as pleasant, even blissful (Cheyne, Rueffer, and Newby-Clark 1999; Hufford 1982; Sherwood 2002; Terrillon and Marques-Bonham 2001). Emotions of joy or contentment contrast sharply with the sense of dread and awareness of an evil presence that accompany the typical night-mare, but both experiences are aspects of sleep paralysis (Davies 2003). Examples of out-of-body experiences are described by physicists Jean-Christophe Terrillon and Sirley Marques-Bonham:

> In the case of proprioceptive hallucinations, the individual feels that he, or part of himself, is at a different location from the physical body: he might feel phantom limbs or he has the subjective experience of slipping away from the physical body in what appears to be a phantom body.

Subjective experiences of floating, rising, and occasionally rolling also occur. In addition, when experiencing an autoscopic hallucination, the proprioceptive hallucination is coupled with visual hallucinations: the individual, while in a floating state, can see the actual room, and eventually his physical body lying motionless on the bed. Or he can see a fictitious, dream-like environment characterized by vivid imagery, or even what seems to be a superposition of both the physical world and a dreamlike world. In all three cases he has a subjective experience of awareness and his experience is perceived to be real. (Terrillon and Marques-Bonham 2001, 108)

Because of the potential to have a transformative experience, there are occasionally Internet discussions about the use of sleep paralysis to produce out-of-body experiences: "There are some folks in this group who actually try to bring on [sleep paralysis] episodes who think it is a gateway to [out-of-body experiences], and others who are convinced that they are being visited by entities or beings from other dimensions. . . . The thought of wanting to have a [sleep paralysis] episode seems pretty crazy to me since my own episodes have been so terrifying" (Internet posting, ASP-L). A writer on another forum is blunter in responding to a request for sleep-paralysis-inducing techniques: "Put yourself under extreme stress all the time. I suggest being a substitute teacher by day, and moonlighting as an air-traffic controller. Seriously, sleep paralysis can be really terrifying. You'd do well to avoid inducing it on purpose" (Internet posting, www.abovetopsecret.com). Despite these warnings, there are people who intentionally induce sleep paralysis in order to have paranormal experiences. Techniques for using sleep paralysis as a "gateway" to the out-of-body state are shared on listservs, and the ability to take advantage of this sleep phenomenon is considered a gift by those who are able to overcome the terror (Proud 2009). This desire to transform sleep paralysis in order to cultivate positive experiences has created something of a cottage industry on the Internet. There are several Web sites that promise to disclose the secrets to "unlocking the potential of sleep paralysis" (for a fee). The following is representative of what is available:

Pay close attention to what I'm about to tell you, or run the risk of ending up like the majority of other sleep paralysis sufferers out there, who become cursed by this condition for their entire lives. Don't say I didn't warn you. Wouldn't it be great to be able to stop these disturbing sleep paralysis episodes? To banish that evil old hag forever? Furthermore, imagine not just being able to stop them, but imagine learning how to actually enjoy them, and even induce them for your own entertainment. . . . I used to experience the evil presence. I used to feel my body turning hard like stone. I used to have terrifying monsters haunt me in the night. I used to hear a loud buzzing noise in my head. I used to feel a smothering and crushing sensation. I used to be sexually violated by unknown beings. I used to be afraid of dying when I closed my eyes at night. I used to think there was no escape. That is of course, until I developed sleep paralysis mastery.

Near-Death Experiences

Although the vast majority of sleep paralysis experiences are extremely disturbing, if not terrifying, there are clearly instances that provide reassurance and even positive transformation. One situation in which dissociation from the physical body can be accompanied by a euphoric or transcendental sensation is when a person is close to death. Raymond Moody introduced the term "near-death experience" in his 1975 book *Life after Life,* which was the first work to compile survivor anecdotes and bring the concept into the medical and popular literature.

> A man is dying and, as he reaches the point of greatest physical distress, he hears himself pronounced dead by his doctor. He begins to hear an uncomfortable noise, a loud ringing or buzzing, and at the same time feels himself moving very rapidly through a long dark tunnel. After this, he suddenly finds himself outside of his own physical body, but still in the immediate physical environment, and he sees his own body from a distance, as though he is a spectator. He watches the resuscitation attempt from this unusual vantage point and is in a state of emotional upheaval. (Moody 1975, 11)

The shared features are obvious: the initial ringing/buzzing sound, the tunnel, autoscopic and proprioceptive sensations. Terrillon and Marques-Bonham note other elements common to some sleep paralysis episodes and some near-death experiences, such as "a feeling of peace and ineffability, vivid and beautiful landscapes, a light that appears at the end of the tunnel and that is bright but does not hurt the eyes" (2001, 111). Like the night-mare, these types of near-death experiences are reported across a variety of cultural settings. As an Inuit woman explains, "It is like that for some people. They can see their body when they are sleeping. My husband almost died. When he woke up he said he had been dreaming. His *tarniq* [soul] was up above his body. When it went back down to his body he woke up. He said he regretted waking up because his *tarniq* had started to ascend" (Kolb and Law 2001, 194).

Although there are common themes, there are also reported differences in the features of near-death experiences from different cultures. An Australian research team of psychiatrists and social workers analyzed narratives of near-death experiences from around the world and found that, while there is acceptance of being "dead" and, hence, estranged from the body, the transcendence of the Western European model is not as prominent in narratives from other cultures. Near-death experiences reported across Africa and in China, India, and Thailand, for example, had "more pragmatic themes such as the offering of food, being sent back because of errors, and a greater focus on good and evil. Meeting deceased relatives was also more common" (Belanti, Perera, and Jagadheesan 2008, 130). The researchers conclude that variability across cultures is most likely due to the interpretation and verbalizing of esoteric events through the filters of language, cultural experiences, religion, and education.[14]

Terrillon and Marques-Bonham suggest that there is an interesting association between the out-of-body experiences that can occur during sleep paralysis and (in what may at first seem to be a completely different circumstance) the traditional ability of shamans to leave their body at will and explore other realms of existence. "In . . . visionary states, the shaman is open to contact with animal allies and spirit helpers. Or the wizard may leave his or her body behind like a husk while the disincarnate soul journeys to the celestial realms above or the underworld of disease and death" (Halifax 1991, 18–19). According to this hypothesis, shamans have learned to control their out-of-body experiences and do not consider sleep paralysis to be an unwanted state of terror.

Neurologist Kevin Nelson and his research team at the University of Kentucky study the links among out-of-body experiences, sleep paralysis, and near-death experiences, and they conclude that some people's brains may be predisposed to these types of events.[15] An out-of-body experience is statistically as likely to occur during a near-death experience as it is to occur during sleep paralysis. "We found it surprising that out-of-body experience with sleep transition seemed very much like out-of-body experience during near-death" (University of Kentucky 2007). In their interview study with fifty-five people who had each had a near-death experience, the researchers noted that those who had an accompanying out-of-body experience were more likely to have experienced sleep paralysis than the age- and gender-matched control subjects. Nelson and colleagues suggest that, during a medical crisis, muscle paralysis combined with an out-of-body experience could show many of the major features of a near-death experience, including disassociation from the physical body, euphoria, and transcendental or mystical elements. This finding supports the idea that out-of-body experiences are an expression of arousal in near-death experiences and sleep paralysis. Almost all of the near-death subjects reported having sleep paralysis: "The strong association of sleep paralysis with out-of-body experiences in the near-death experience subject is curious and unexplained. However, persons with near-death experiences appear to have an arousal system predisposed to both REM intrusion and out-of-body experiences" (University of Kentucky 2007). Nelson and his research team explain that sensations related to sleep paralysis possess characteristics that are easily transformed into features of near-death experiences, such as the sensed presence of an entity or floating out of the body. Near-death experiences are also recalled with an intense sense of reality and lack the bizarre characteristics of dreams. The researchers hypothesize that REM intrusion could form the basis of subjective phenomena strikingly similar to near-death experiences (Nelson, Mattingly, and Schmitt 2007). Ironically, while laboratory sleep research has thus made an enormous contribution to the scientific understanding of anomalous experiences, in addition to the comprehension of the night-mare's core features, it has simultaneously corroborated thousands of years of empirical evidence from night-mare sufferers.

5

The Night-mare, Traditional Hmong Culture, and Sudden Death

"Hmong refugees do not seek new lives, they seek the same lives in a new location, and where possible they use their new opportunities to bolster preexisting social conceptions."

—Nancy Donnelly (1994, 184)

Sudden Death and the Night-mare: Is There a Connection?

Since the first reported case, which occurred in 1977, more than 117 Southeast Asians in the United States have died from the disorder that is now known as SUNDS, the Sudden Unexpected Nocturnal Death Syndrome. The sudden deaths have had an unusually high incidence rate among Laotians, particularly Hmong refugees.[1] All but one of the victims have been men; their median age is thirty-three; and the median length of time that they lived in the United States before their death is seventeen months (Parrish 1988). No one had complained of illness or discomfort before going to bed; all were considered by family members to have been in good health. Occasionally, the deaths were witnessed by a relative who had been awakened by the sound of gasping or moaning, but the sleeper would die within a minute or two. Most victims, however, were unresponsive when they were found and could not be revived. The deaths occurred with alarming frequency; at their peak in 1981–82, the rate of death from SUNDS among twenty-five- to forty-four-year-old Hmong men was 92 per 100,000 (Baron and Kirschner 1983), a figure equivalent to the combined rate of the five leading causes of natural death among men in the United States in the same age group.

Despite numerous studies of SUNDS—exploring such diverse but potentially relevant issues as electrolytes and circadian cycles (Holtan et al. 1984), genetics (Marshall 1981; Munger and Hurlich 1981),[2] heart disease (Kirschner, Eckner, and Baron 1986; Otto et al. 1984), mental health (Westermeyer 1981), metabolic problems (Bliatout 1982), nutrition (American Refugee Committee 1989), sleep apnea (Holtan et al. 1984), and toxicology (Bissinger 1981; Bliatout 1982; Holtan et al. 1984; Pyle 1981)—medical scientists were not able to determine exactly what was causing the sudden nocturnal deaths. The most plausible of the hypotheses implicated a problem with the heart's electrical conduction system, but a 1988 report from the Centers for Disease Control underscored the limitations of even this possibility: "Only at night, in times of unusual stress, and possibly in conjunction with other, as yet undefined, factors are these people at risk of developing abnormal electrical impulses in the heart that result in ventricular fibrillation and sudden death" (Parrish 1988).

In the summer of 1984, a group of epidemiologists gathered at the St. Paul-Ramsey Medical Center (now Regions Hospital) in Minnesota to propose methods for studying SUNDS and to formulate recommendations for public health officials responding to the crisis. People at high risk for SUNDS were defined as "those who fit the demographic characteristics and have one of the following signs or three of the following symptoms":

SIGNS

1. breathing pauses in sleep
2. seizures or muscle spasms during sleep
3. loud snoring, gasping, or choking sounds during sleep
4. cyanosis during sleep
5. unarousability from sleep

SYMPTOMS

1. a sense of panic or extreme fear
2. paralysis (partial or complete)
3. a sense of pressure on the chest
4. a sense that there is an alien being (animal, human, or spirit) in the room
5. a disturbance in sensation (auditory, visual, or tactile) (Holtan et al. 1984, 11)

The symptoms of SUNDS-related events clearly mirror the features of the night-mare as it has been known across cultures and throughout history. The signs are more difficult to interpret, but interrupted breathing and choking sounds might be traditionally viewed as the consequence of an attack by a pressing spirit. Muscle spasms, cyanosis (skin taking on a bluish color due to insufficient oxygen in the blood), and "unarousability" are not consistent with a typical night-mare attack and may more accurately reflect a later stage of SUNDS itself.

The parallels between epidemiologist-reported symptoms and those experienced by night-mare sufferers themselves prompt a critical question: Does the existence of a distinctive symptom constellation suggest a link between the night-mare encounter and Hmong SUNDS, or is it simply an artifact of misinterpretation on the part of scientists unfamiliar with the characteristics and distribution of the night-mare? At a meeting of the epidemiology discussion group of the SUNDS Planning Project, one researcher suggested that "those persons who have described the 'spirit or figure pressing against the chest' at night

during sleep making breathing difficult would be productive persons to interview. This complaint might even be considered as a type of 'marker' for future
studies or even intervention trials" (Holtan 1984). If there is a connection
between the deaths and the ongoing and universal night-mare tradition, why
did SUNDS predominantly affect Laotian Hmong men? Why did most deaths
occur within two years of relocation to the United States, and why did the deaths
then taper off and stop? Because of my training in traditional belief and narrative, my inclination was to turn to those most directly affected—the Hmong
immigrants themselves—for answers.[3]

As a first step in exploring a possible connection between the night-mare
and the sudden deaths, I set out to learn whether there was in fact a living tradition of a nocturnal pressing spirit among Hmong immigrants. I selected the
city of Stockton, a trade and agricultural center sixty-five miles east of San
Francisco in California's Central Valley, as the site of my field research.[4] I conducted fieldwork over a period of fourteen months, interviewing 118 Hmong
men and women and speaking informally with scores of others. I visited community centers and clinics, observed shamanic ceremonies, and attended New
Year celebrations. I am still surprised at the degree of access I was granted and
how warmly I was received (after people were reassured that I had no ties to welfare or other government agencies). Despite the tragic focus of my research,
Hmong men and women were remarkably welcoming, open, and eager to share
their experiences with me and, by extension, other Americans.

The Night-mare and Traditional Hmong Religion:
Animism, Ancestor Worship, and Shamanism

In order to begin to understand the impact of SUNDS on Hmong men and
women in communities in the United States, it is important to have at least
some background understanding of traditional Hmong culture. Rather than
attempt to present an ethnography of the Laotian Hmong, I will instead include
brief summaries of aspects of Hmong culture and history that illuminate the
night-mare traditions and experiences that were recounted to me. These snap-
shot descriptions are generalizations; as with all groups, not every Hmong man
or woman I spoke with participates equally in the beliefs and behaviors associated with the "Hmong culture" with which they formally identify themselves.

There has been much speculation about the geographic origins of the Hmong
people,[5] but, regardless of their prehistory, they were living in settlements in
the plains along China's Yellow River by 3,000 BCE. Over the next few millennia,
they were constantly driven southward by sustained ethnic persecution, including efforts at forced assimilation under Chinese rule (Chiu 2004). In the nineteenth century, the Hmong emigrated south and southwest out of China, entering
into what we now know as Vietnam, then Laos, and eventually Thailand. (Almost

all of the Hmong immigrants to the United States are from Laos, officially the Lao People's Democratic Republic.)

The Hmong are not a homogeneous group, and there is no standardized code of Laotian Hmong religious practice. There are, in fact, many dissimilarities, some originating in regional differences. Despite the variations, however, broad outlines of the traditional Hmong belief system remain distinct, combining beliefs and practices of animism, ancestor worship, and shamanism (Her 2005).

Animism

Animism is the belief that spirits and spiritual forces inhabit the natural universe. Trees, mountains, rivers, rocks, and lightning are all animated by distinctive beings, and most animals are considered kindred creatures who share and exchange souls with humans. Protective ancestor spirits also continue to interact with their living descendants. Most nature spirits have no interest in human affairs unless they are offended in some way, but untamed evil spirits, which often lurk in uninhabited areas, can attack people and cause misfortune, illness, or death (Cha 2003). The traditional Hmong nocturnal pressing spirit, *dab tsog* (pronounced "da cho"), is one of these wild spirits. *Dab* is the Hmong word for "spirit," and it is often used in the sense of an evil spirit; *tsog* is the specific name of the night-mare spirit. Another common term to denote a night-mare attack is *tsog tsuam* (pronounced "cho chua"); *tsuam* means "to crush, to press, or to smother" (Heimbach 1979). In Laos, *dab tsog* often make their homes in caverns. Hmong girls and women avoid going into or near caves because of the danger that *dab tsog* will rape them. When *dab tsog* assaults a woman, she becomes infertile; if she is pregnant at the time of the attack, she will miscarry.[6] In my interviews with Hmong men and women, however, it became clear that *dab tsog* is notorious for visiting sleepers in the night, sitting or lying upon them, pressing down and squeezing them tightly, preventing their movement, and trying to suffocate them.

Ancestor Worship

In the traditional Hmong religion, ancestor worship is based on the interdependence between deceased forebears and their living offspring. Ancestors' spirits continue to influence the daily lives and welfare of their descendants, who offer food and observe the proper rituals to ensure that the ancestors are remembered and worshipped. At death, individuals' souls are guided back to the land of their ancestors, so it is critical that the progenitors' spirits be kept satisfied. The human body hosts a set of (typically three) souls: one ordinarily accompanies the body, one wanders (this is the soul that causes people to dream when they sleep), and one protects its owner from harm. A person is healthy when all of the souls are within the body, living harmoniously together. Illness is produced when a soul leaves the body of its own will[7] or is disturbed or abducted by a malevolent spirit. The best method to avoid these evil spirits is the proper care of ancestor spirits, who protect their living descendants. When a person dies, the first soul remains with the body at the grave site, the second soul returns to live with his or her descendants as an ancestor spirit, and the third may be reincarnated (either as a human being, animal, or object).

Shamanism

Since ordinary people cannot see or communicate with the spirits, it is up to a shaman, with his (or, less commonly, her) extraordinary powers, to intercede and act as an ambassador from our world to the other. Each shaman works with a *neeb* (pronounced "neng"), a special healing spirit.

The *ua neeb* ritual, with its many variations, represents the culmination of a Hmong shaman's healing power (Thao 1986). While in a trance, a shaman searches for an individual's lost soul with the help of his *neeb;* he sits and occasionally jumps or bounces on a bench (or "horse"), his eyes are covered by a black cloth, and an assistant rhythmically beats a gong. After arriving in the spirit world, the shaman tries to discover both the cause of the illness (most frequently soul loss, an offended ancestor spirit, an angered nature spirit, or a malicious untamed evil spirit) and what can be done to rectify the situation (often an animal sacrifice).

Stalking the Hmong Night-mare

I began my research by interviewing Hmong men and women about potential night-mare encounters, but I was careful to base my initial questions on generic night-mare characteristics (e.g., "Did you ever wake up during the night and realize that you were unable to move or speak?"). Only later in the interview did I ask for definitions of emic night-mare terms (e.g., "What is *dab tsog?*"). In this way, I hoped to separate my questions about the experience of sleep paralysis from those related to specific cultural beliefs.[8] I was surprised to find not only that 58 percent of the people I interviewed had experienced at least one night-mare, but that 97 percent of interviewees were familiar with *dab tsog* or *tsog tsuam.* The Hmong night-mare was clearly a collective tradition.

The Night-mare in Traditional Context: Dab Tsog in Laos

One of the first narratives of a night-mare attack was retold to me by Jia Neng Her,[9] a forty-five-year-old man who had come to the United States in 1988 after thirteen years in a Thai refugee camp. Her was a shaman, as was his father. He experienced three or four night-mares in Laos, beginning in 1962.

> The first *dab tsog* that came to me, I remember that I was in the jungle. It
> happened more when I was not at home, when I was sleeping in the

jungle. I was lying on my back and I felt that someone was coming and lying down beside me. Then someone was lying on top of me. It felt so heavy. I felt so scared. I tried for a long time to move. After a long time, I could move. I could see no one. My friend that was next to me was still asleep. But *dab tsog* was not there anymore.

Her describes the classic night-mare features: paralysis, pressure on the chest, lying in a supine position, sensing a presence, and extreme fear. A traditional Hmong explanation for this type of *dab tsog* attack is that the area of the jungle that Her was sleeping in was inhabited by untamed evil spirits. Her's experience also fits the cross-cultural pattern of night-mares that occur in relation to sleep disruptions (e.g., sleeping in an unfamiliar area or bed, sleeping at an unusual time).

Her continued his account with a description of the traditional intervention that takes place after a person has experienced a series of *dab tsog* attacks: "When someone has *dab tsog* come to them, they need a shaman. The shaman can find out why *dab tsog* is coming and they can take *dab tsog* away. They also have something for the person to wear. Usually they have the twisted metal for the neck, but sometimes, not a lot, for the arm or ankle." This twisted metal necklace is made of three entwined cords of silver, copper, and iron. Her explained to me that the neck-ring is worn as protection from evil spirits; it confines the soul to the body and thus prevents the soul's wandering or being scared away by a malicious spirit. It also alters the appearance of the victim so that *dab tsog* cannot locate him or her, and, being made of iron, it repels *dab tsog*. The ritual object was not used in isolation, however; the shaman played an important role in preventing (repeated) evil spirit attacks.

It doesn't matter if you are a man or woman—[*dab tsog*] happens the same to both. Human beings have spirits also—souls—and every year the shaman has to call our own spirit to stay with our body. We call this *hu plig* [pronounced "hoo plee"]. If the shaman is doing this about every year, then most people will not have *dab tsog*. But whoever did not have the shaman call their spirit to come to their body, then their own spirit is far away from them, and *dab tsog* can catch that person. If a person's soul is unhappy and far away, *dab tsog* can come close to them.

Another representative Laotian night-mare attack was recounted for me by Chue Lor, a fifty-eight-year-old Hmong man who arrived in the United States in 1979 after spending six months in a Thai refugee camp. He experienced his first of four night-mares, which he referred to as *tsog tsuam,* at the age of nineteen or twenty. Lor remembers that he was not feeling well at the time of the first attack, and had gone to bed earlier in the evening than usual. Although his encounter took place more than thirty-five years before our interview, Lor's narrative conveys the immediacy typical of first-person retellings of night-mare attacks.

> I was in my bed at night. There were people at the other end of the house and I could hear them talking. They were still talking outside. I heard everything. But I knew that someone else was there. Suddenly there comes a huge body, it looked like—like a big stuffed animal they sell here. It was over me—on my body—and I had to fight my way out of that. I couldn't move—I couldn't talk at all. I couldn't even yell, "No!" By the time it was over, I remember, there were four other people inside and they said, "You made all this noise." I was trying to fight myself against that and it was very, very, very scary. That particular spirit was big, black, hairy. Big teeth. Big eyes. I was very, very scared.

Lor's description includes an element that is present in almost every Hmong night-mare narrative: the realistic perception of the environment. People from different ethnic backgrounds who have shared their night-mare experiences with me invariably and spontaneously emphasize that they were not asleep during the encounter. There seems to be a universal need to emphasize this distinction between night-mares and dreams. As Lor describes, "There were people at the other end of the house and I could hear them talking." The juxtaposition of ordinary aspects of waking life with the shock of the appearance of unearthly elements appears to intensify the night-mare's impact (not only on Hmong men and women who practice their traditional religion, but also on people without animist beliefs). The intrusion of a supranormal figure into the mundane world heightens the reality of the terrifying visitor. I continued the interview by asking, "What position were you sleeping in?"

> I was on my back. I could hear the other people talking, but I couldn't yell to them to help me. I couldn't breathe, I couldn't even move. And so, finally, finally—I still remember, because I was so scared—the way that I got out of it was I used one of my fingers to poke one of his eyes. And the moment that he—he or she, whatever—that thing got off of me, that's when I woke up. I told everyone there and then, immediately, and they brought me a knife to put under my pillow when I slept. The next day my father called a shaman and he performed a ritual, and that was it—that was the end of it.

Lor's efforts to poke the spirit with his finger recall the widespread remedy of focusing intently on one small movement to end a night-mare attack (e.g., wiggling a finger or toe, making the sign of the cross with one's tongue). Sleeping with a knife under the pillow is a common night-mare preventive cross-culturally (and iron is used to ward off evil spirits in many traditions).

It was becoming clear from my interviews that *dab tsog* attacks shared characteristics of cross-cultural night-mare traditions. How, then, could this relatively common experience be considered potentially lethal?

LOR: When the spirit comes, it presses down—pushes down on you. You are scared of moving. You feel so scared, like you could die. You feel that if it doesn't stop, you will die. But I was okay. I didn't move, and after a while it went away.

ADLER: Can *tsog tsuam* actually kill people, or does it just frighten you and make you feel that you might die?

LOR: It always scares you and you feel that you will die. Usually people don't die the first time. After it happens once or twice, you go to a shaman and they help you. If it happens a few times and a shaman doesn't help you to find out why, then the spirit may be very angry and *tsog tsuam* can kill you.

How is it that *tsog tsuam* gains access to human beings? Lor explains: "When the Hmong don't worship properly, do not perform the religious ritual properly or forget to sacrifice or whatever, then the ancestor spirits or the village spirits do not want to guard them. That's why the evil spirit is able to come and get them." He later clarified that, although evil spirits have tremendous innate power to afflict human beings, it is primarily in the absence of ancestor spirits that they are able to exercise their malevolent will.

I was beginning to understand how SUNDS was conceptualized as a *dab tsog* attack, but, since both men and women were visited by *dab tsog* (in equal numbers among the people I spoke with), it was not clear how people accounted for the fact that only one woman had died of SUNDS. Lor explains that *dab tsog* encounters also have gender-specific effects: "It happens to both men and women, but the problem for women is that if the shaman can't help her, or if you can't find a shaman right away, then the woman will not be pregnant anymore. The spirit will be just like her boyfriend or something like that." *Dab tsog* attacks on women are not thought to have the same lethal potential as those perpetrated on men.[10] The gender dichotomy that characterizes Hmong culture in Laos appears to play a role in Hmong interpretation of the causes of *dab tsog* attacks. Traditionally, Hmong gender roles are hierarchically arranged and expressed through a clear division of tasks: "The husband has responsibility to know the traditions, the customs, the oral history, the lineage, the details of the group's rituals, to interact with others, to make the major decisions about the future of the family. The wife takes care of the money, raises the children, and in Laos, did much of the daily work, including field work, making clothes, cooking, and tending livestock" (Vang and Lewis 1984, 12). Anthropologist Nancy Donnelly, who conducted ethnographic research in Seattle's Hmong community during the 1980s, explains that, as in other cultures, Hmong men and women maintain "informational blind spots" (1994, 79). Hmong women do not seem to have any systematic knowledge of men's ritual roles. "Most of my subjects were afraid of spirits but drew a blank when asked about how beliefs fit together" (Donnelly 1994, 86). According to Lor, this lack of familiarity with and responsibility for religious tasks is protective for women.

Hmong Refugees: From Laos, through Thailand, to the United States

In 1961, many Laotian Hmong joined together under the command of General Vang Pao to fight the Pathet Lao troops and the North Vietnamese army. Urged by the Royal Lao government and funded by the United States Central Intelligence Agency, Hmong men served as soldiers, pilots, and navigators; their familiarity with the mountainous terrain made them excellent scouts and guerrilla fighters. Despite their efforts, however, the war was lost in April 1975. Nearly one-third of the Laotian Hmong population lost their lives—a casualty rate proportionally ten times higher than that of Americans who fought in the Vietnam War (Cerquone 1986). Although Hmong men had served on both sides, all Laotian Hmong became the target of communist hostility after Vientiane fell to the Pathet Lao. Most Hmong had hoped to stay in the country that they had fought so fiercely to defend, but it soon became clear that rumored Pathet Lao threats of a Hmong genocide were accurate. In 1975, a writer for the *Khaosan Pathet Lao,* the newspaper of the Laotian Communist Party, confirmed, "We must eradicate the [Hmong] minority completely" (Dao 1982, 13). Tens of thousands of Hmong men and women who were not able to escape suffered torture and death in "seminar" camps, but the majority fled Laos. The harrowing nighttime escapes through jungle and across the Mekong River were compounded by Pathet Lao ambush patrols, as well as starvation, disease, and drownings. Those who managed to reach Thailand sought asylum in refugee camps that were plagued by safety, sanitation, and other health problems (Cerquone 1986). The Thai government attempted to resettle many of the Hmong who had been living in refugee camps, but preparatory efforts were minimal and thousands of Hmong departed for new countries—primarily the United States—with only the most perfunctory arrangements.

The Hmong people who fled Laos left behind a homeland ravaged by war, but in their transition to the United States, they were met with new and often unanticipated problems. Hmong immigrants found themselves in a place where their skills, language, and religion were decontextualized and where their previous social support system was dismantled. When the first refugees began arriving in 1975, resettlement officials implemented a plan to avoid "overburdening" individual communities with new immigrants. Under a short-sighted federal "scattering" policy, families were randomly dispersed, without regard to clan affiliation or the extended families that had been an important source of emotional and economic support in Laos (Westermeyer 1987). John Finck, of the

Rhode Island Office of Refugee Resettlement, explained that the Hmong were spread "like a thin layer of butter throughout the country so they'd disappear" (Morin 1983). Small, fractured groups were directed to fifty-three cities in twenty-five states; families were sent wherever a church group or local community would sponsor them (Viviano 1986). As soon as they had gathered the resources to rejoin their families, clans, and friends, though, many Hmong left their initial resettlement communities as part of a "secondary migration." The three major destinations for this self-directed move were California, Wisconsin, and Minnesota. (Minneapolis-St. Paul is now home to the largest single community of Hmong in the world.) Unfortunately, the initial phase of the secondary migration yielded disappointing results. Although the Hmong exodus was a tribute to human resourcefulness and resulted in reuniting long-separated families, a closer look revealed "up to 90 percent unemployment . . . [and] a high suicide rate" (Thompson 1986, 48).

Difficulties in learning a new language and finding employment may not be unique to Hmong refugees,[11] but the constellation of issues that includes changing gender and generational roles, survivor guilt, trauma-induced emotional and psychological disorders, and the conflict between a traditional religion and Christianity is not shared by all immigrants to the United States. In addition, the skills essential to life in highland Laos, such as farming and hunting, were for the most part not easily transferred to the U.S. economy.[12] The majority of Hmong immigrants initially had no choice but to rely on public assistance funds. Chong Sao Yang, a sixty-two-year-old former farmer and soldier who resettled in San Diego, California, expresses a common sentiment:

> In our old country, whatever we had was made or brought in by our own hands. We are not born on earth to have somebody give us food. Here, I'm sure we're going to starve, because since our arrival there is no penny I can get that is money I earn from work. I've been trying very hard to learn English, and at the same time look for a job. But no matter what kind of job, even a job to clean people's toilets, still people don't trust you or offer you such work. I'm not even worth as much as a dog's stool. Talking about this, I want to die right here so I won't see my future. (Whitman 1987, 18)

In addition to language and employment issues created by the transition to the United States, resettlement brought with it a series of challenges to the traditional Hmong patriarchal system (Lee 1994–95; Meredith and Rowe 1986). Changes were occurring that threatened the status of the traditional male role (Faderman and Xiong 1998; Fadiman 1997); Hmong men were no longer the sole supporters of their families. Unable to find jobs, they were forced to accept the economic gains of their wives' and daughters' embroidery. Hmong men, traditionally responsible for conducting all formal communication outside the family, were unable to speak, read, or write English. Changes in generational roles also altered the traditional Hmong social hierarchy. Historically, relationships of respect privileged elders, but in the United States, Hmong girls and boys attended school and not only learned English and other subjects and skills completely unknown to their parents, but also became acculturated much more quickly than men and women of older generations (Kaiser 2004–05).

Anthropologists Jacques Lemoine and Christine Mougne hypothesize that the difficulties that Hmong men, in particular, experienced often resulted in loss of self-respect, a feeling of lack of control over their own lives, severe depression, and a loss of will to live under such anxious circumstances (1983). Anthropologist Joseph Tobin and social worker Joan Friedman apply insights gained from studies of World War II Holocaust survivors to the plight of Hmong refugees and focus on "survivor stress," the outcome of conflicting feelings of relief at having reached asylum and sorrow over the loss of loved ones (1983). The challenges of resettlement—psychological, social, and economic—form the backdrop against which the American night-mare appeared.

Cultural Representation and Hmong Immigrants

Anthropologist Aihwa Ong writes that "Southeast Asian refugees remain among the most invisible groups in the North American consciousness" (2003, xvi). The Hmong, however, are more widely known in the West than other Southeast Asian ethnic groups, perhaps because of their efforts on behalf of the United States during the war in Vietnam, particularly after it spread to Laos and Cambodia (Hamilton-Merritt 1999). Much more recently, Anne Fadiman's book *The Spirit Catches You and You Fall Down: A Hmong Child, Her American Doctors, and the Collision of Two Cultures* (1997), introduced many North Americans to aspects of traditional Hmong culture. Unfortunately, though, other examples of Hmong visibility have clustered around tragedies such as gang violence, the fatal shooting in 2005 of six white European American hunters in Wisconsin by a Hmong hunter (Miller 2005), and the sudden nocturnal deaths.

Disturbingly, many journalistic accounts have associated SUNDS with the presumed "cultural primitivity" of the Hmong (Ong 2003). Magazine and newspaper articles portray the Hmong as a "Stone Age" people (Shulins 1984), "ruled by superstition and myth" (Carlson 1981), and puzzling "over the tools of the industrial revolution as the rest of America marches into the computer age" (Sherman 1988, 589). "Frozen in time," the Hmong are described as "unable to speak English or read their own language [and struggling] with the simplest parts of modern life—flicking a light switch, turning a faucet" (Donnelly 2005). The image of the primitive and exotic Hmong is disturbingly persistent, if not, given North American biases, surprising. As historian and anthropologist James Clifford writes:

> Whenever marginal peoples come into a historical or ethnographic space
> that has been defined by the Western imagination . . . their distinct

histories quickly vanish. . . . [T]hese suddenly "backward" people no longer invent local futures. What is different about them remains tied to traditional pasts, inherited structures that either resist or yield to the new but cannot produce it. (2002, 5)

In the case of the Hmong refugees, stereotypes constrain still further; rather than being viewed as yielding to the new, the Hmong have been portrayed as stubbornly *resisting* American influence. In 1987, Senator Alan Simpson, then the ranking minority member of the Senate Subcommittee on Immigration and Refugee Affairs, called the Hmong "the most indigestible group in society" (Simpson 1987, 4).[13]

Even Fadiman's best-selling book has been criticized by Hmong-American scholars for her "contextualization through an ethnographic gaze that often renders the Lao Hmong exotic" (Chiu 2004–05, 4) or "idealizes" (Lee 1998) or "romanticizes" them (Yang 1998). The "continued Hmong mythologization" (Chiu 2004–05, 4) does as great a disservice to heterogeneous Hmong culture as the journalistic obsession with the "primitive." It is fitting, therefore, that the same sudden geographic proximity that conveniently affords reporters views of an "exotic" population also provides opportunities for the subjects of this journalistic gaze to critique their observers. When an article in the *New York Times* called the Hmong "the most primitive refugee group in America" (Mydans 1990), a reader responded, "[E]vidently we were not too primitive to fight as proxies for the United States troops in the war in Laos" (Herr 1990).

The stereotypes of the Hmong as primitive and "other" also contributed to sensationalized portrayals of their susceptibility to disease. Like other Southeast Asian refugees,[14] the Hmong were represented as vulnerable—that is, culturally susceptible—to mysterious illnesses impenetrable to modern medicine. For example, when the nighttime pattern of SUNDS became known, some journalists and scientists became morbidly fascinated by the prospect of lethal dreams.

Did a palm tree's fronds turn into threatening fingers? Did a forest move and march with the implacability of the tide? Did a rose stretch on its stalk and throttle the sleeper? Or did a gasoline hose curl and crush like a python? Was one of the dreamers pinned by a perambulating postbox? Or stabbed by scissors run amok? Whatever caused the Laotians' deaths is beyond autopsy; it defies dissection. (*New York Times*, June 7, 1981)

In this national atmosphere of exoticizing the Hmong refugees, I wanted to represent faithfully the views of the people I spoke with regarding SUNDS and also present their understandings in a way that would allow other Americans to relate to their experiences. The Hmong night-mare is, of course, only one example of a universal tradition—albeit one with which North Americans, as a consequence of war and politics, have come into closer contact. Surely the many examples of fractured night-mare traditions from around the world that have survived their original cultural contexts were once as vital and finely articulated as those we find in contemporary Hmong settings.

The Relocated Night-mare: *Dab Tsog* in the United States

Traditional Hmong Religion

Hmong men and women told me that they had feared that the ancestor spirits who protected them from harm in Laos would be unable to travel across the ocean to the United States and thus would leave them vulnerable to spiritual dangers. Nevertheless, the refugees took solace in the conviction that the myriad evil spirits that had threatened Hmong well-being in Southeast Asia would also be prevented from following them to their new home. It soon became frighteningly apparent, though, that *dab tsog* had made the journey to North America, as well.

Tobin and Friedman present the case of Vang Xiong, a twenty-two-year-old Hmong man who resettled in Chicago in 1980 and "who experienced what the Hmong call a spirit problem, and what we call an acute mental health crisis, shortly after his arrival in America." The authors use the case "to document the presence in a Southeast Asian refugee of the kind of survivor guilt previously reported chiefly in World War II Holocaust survivors" (1983, 439). Xiong and his family seemed to do well for the first few months in Chicago, but the difficulties began after they moved into a new apartment.

> The first night he woke suddenly, short of breath, from a dream in which a cat was sitting on his chest. The second night, the room suddenly grew darker, and a figure, like a large black dog, came to his bed and sat on his chest. He could not push the dog off and he grew quickly and dangerously short of breath. The third night, a tall, white-skinned female spirit came into his bedroom from the kitchen and lay on top of him. Her weight made it increasingly difficult for him to breathe. . . . He attempted to turn onto his side, but found he was pinned down. After fifteen minutes, the spirit left him. (Tobin and Friedman 1983, 440)

Xiong fortunately did not suffer cardiac arrest during sleep, but, as Tobin and Friedman explain, his age and background, as well as the symptoms of his sleep disturbance, were consistent with those of many SUNDS victims.[15]

Xiong interpreted the experiences as a spirit attack. He consulted a widely respected shaman, Mrs. Thor, who determined that the problem was caused by the previous tenants' souls, which had been left behind after the tenants' abrupt departure. She then performed a ritual to encourage the spirits to move on.

Xiong explained that similar spirit encounters had been experienced by him and his brother in Laos:

> We are susceptible to such attacks because we didn't follow all of the mourning rituals we should have when our parents died. Because we didn't properly honor their memories we have lost contact with their spirits, and thus we are left with no one to protect us from evil spirits. I had hoped flying so far in a plane to come to America would protect me, but it turns out spirits can follow even this far. (Tobin and Friedman 1983, 444)

A similar, but more detailed, explanation is offered by another Hmong immigrant that I interviewed, Chia Vue. This forty-nine-year-old man had left Laos in 1980 and, after living in a Thai refugee camp for one year, came to the United States. He had two episodes of *tsog tsuam* during his first two years of resettlement. Vue is one of very few people who used the English word *nightmare* to label his *tsog tsuam* experiences. His usage parallels my own in adopting the historical term; in Vue's narrative, *nightmare* and *tsog tsuam* refer to the same event.

After finally arriving in the United States, Vue constantly worried about his family and his own livelihood. On the night of his first *tsog tsuam* encounter, he was preoccupied with troubling thoughts.

> I remember a few months after I first came here—I was asleep. I turned out the light and everything, but I kind of think about, think about, think about, and then—all of a sudden, I felt that—I cannot move. I just feel it, but I don't see anything, but I—then I tried to move my hand, but I cannot move my hand. I keep trying, but I cannot move myself. I know it is *tsog tsuam*. I am so scared. I can hardly breathe. I think, "Who will help me? What if I die?"

The emotional stress and preoccupation with worrisome thoughts ("think about, think about, think about") that precede Vue's attack are familiar from cross-cultural examples of predisposing factors. Mental exhaustion was also part of Vue's second assault.

> I was sort of sleeping. My eyes were still open and I was still seeing. I felt that I could—could not move. It's like a ghost putting pressure on you. Something like that. I saw someone come to me and start pushing me. I could not breathe, I could not talk, I could not yell. But I can still see the TV, I can still see the light. Like, in my brain, I'm saying, "Move! Move!" but my body cannot. I try—keep trying to move. I am so frightened. I feel I am alone. But I'm still trying to move—kick this spirit off of me. Finally, I can move my legs, and then my arms. Right away, I can move my whole body—and then the spirit runs away.

Except for small contextualizing details ("I can still see the TV"), Vue's post-resettlement night-mare experience is indistinguishable from *dab tsog* attacks in Laos. Given this similarity, I needed to learn what was considered so different about night-mare experiences in the new context of the United States that could allow for a connection between *dab tsog* attacks and SUNDS to be made. I began to focus on any comments regarding death and dying that participants spontaneously included in their narratives. For example:

VUE: During his lifetime, the person who died of SUNDS usually has at least two night-mares before it really becomes serious.

ADLER: Why, after two non-fatal attacks, would it become so much worse?

VUE: It is believed that once you have one of those night-mares—you are visited by one of the *dab tsog* evil spirits—once you are seen by one of those evil spirits, often they will come back to you, until you have the worst night-mare and probably die.

According to Vue's interpretation, *tsog tsuam* attacks are rarely, if ever, fatal on the first encounter. Typically, the lethal potential is realized only after a Hmong man has been given time to rectify a situation but is unable or chooses not to satisfy the attacking spirit. Vue thus sees a direct connection between Hmong night-mares and SUNDS.

Interestingly, Vue also believes that there is a hereditary component of the sudden deaths, an idea that has also been the focus of much scientific SUNDS research. "If my relative did not have any nightmares, it is likely that I won't have any nightmares; but if my relative used to have nightmares and died in his sleep, it is more likely that it will happen to me." Despite his belief in the heritable nature of SUNDS, though, Vue says, "There were night-mares [in Laos], but the sudden death was unheard of. It might have happened, but I never heard of it." Indeed, none of the people I interviewed recalled incidents of SUNDS deaths in Laos.[16] This finding, which is also reported in several early newspaper accounts of the "mystery deaths" (e.g., Maxwell 1981b), is, admittedly, problematic. It is difficult to know whether people in isolated mountain communities would be aware of similar deaths in other remote areas.

The last significant factor that Vue helped me understand is the reason for people's intense fear of the *dab tsog* attack as retribution—that there is a causal relationship between failing to perform traditional Hmong rituals and being victimized by an evil spirit.

At least once a year those evil spirits must be fed. If someone forgets to feed them, then they will come back and disturb you. If you have *tsog tsuam,* the ancestor spirit is supposed to protect you. If you feed the ancestors regularly, then whenever you have *tsog tsuam* the ancestor spirits will protect you. Usually the father, the head-of-household, is responsible for feeding the evil spirits. Women have night-mares, too, but not as often as men. The evil spirit would first attack the head-of-household. Coming to this country, people tend to forget to do the rituals. A lot of people either ignore or forget to practice their religious belief. . . . If you have a night-mare, and the spirit intends to make you die, it will simply take your soul away. . . . Men are the ones who are responsible for feeding both the evil spirits and the ancestor spirits. Since they are not doing their part, it is logical that their soul should be taken away.

Vue's belief in the link between SUNDS and *dab tsog,* and his explanation for the deaths, address the gender distribution. When I asked interviewees why only one woman had died, they replied that she must have been, due to divorce or widow-hood, viewed by *dab tsog* as the head of her household. This association of night-mares and SUNDS was articulated for me directly by several Hmong men and women, and the explanation fits well with the distribution of SUNDS. Only one aspect of SUNDS remained unaccounted for in the Hmong interpretations: If there was a connection between *dab tsog* and the sudden deaths that was mediated by traditional religious beliefs, how could it affect both animists and Christians?

Hmong Christianity

Hmong immigrants to the United States have experienced a religious transition so extreme that one researcher referred to it as "the spiritual readjustment of a people" (Desan 1983, 45). Hmong men and women who wanted to continue to practice their traditional religion faced a series of daunting obstacles. First, in practical terms, sacrificial animals necessary to "feed the ancestors" were nearly impossible to obtain, and, if acquired, were difficult to sacrifice in the urban environments of many early Hmong communities. The cost of the rituals, which, apart from the animal offering, includes (additional) food and drink for a large gathering, was often prohibitive. Also, many Hmong men and women appropriately feared negative repercussions from their noisy, often protracted rituals (Fadiman 1997). Desan states the problem succinctly: "[F]or a people seeking to maintain harmony with their surroundings, practices incompatible with those surroundings are inadmissible" (1983, 46). Psychiatrist Joseph Westermeyer writes that "many depressed patients were non-Christian animists (i.e., believed in spirits) who had been placed with Christian pastor-sponsors in rural areas. . . . These refugee-sponsor combinations led to numerous cultural, religious, behavioral, and attitudinal conflicts" (1988, 67).

The greatest spiritual transition was Hmong conversion to Christianity. Missionary activity, primarily on the part of the French, led to the conversion of some Hmong while still in Laos, but over two-thirds of the Christian Hmong I interviewed converted after their relocation to the United States. While some Hmong men and women changed religion out of a genuine desire to worship and practice as Christians, there were also those who converted out of a sense of loyalty or obligation to their church sponsors or for a variety of other nonreligious reasons. As is universally true, conversion is not necessarily an accurate gauge of internal conviction. Desan notes, for example, that several hundred Hmong refugees in Philadelphia were associated with various Christian churches, but that the "majority of ministers . . . suggest that most of the refugees attend because of a desire for community, not doctrine" (1983, 48).

According to a Hmong social worker in Stockton, California:

> It's hard to tell how many Hmong are Christian. They are strong, strong believers in their traditional religion. When they adapt to this society, this new lifestyle, their children go to church—but when they come home, they still worship like before. . . . Some people go to church on Sundays, but when they come home, they still have [an ancestor altar] and worship like that.

In fact, many of the Christian Hmong with whom I spoke describe strategies for combining the two religions in order to prevent incurring the wrath of various Hmong spirits. As Dia Cha, an anthropologist at St. Cloud State University in Minnesota, explains: "The Christian messages embraced by some Hmong are not always those espoused by their Western missionaries. Rather, Christian ideas are occasionally modified to fit the Procrustean bed of Hmong cultural expectations, and have come thereby to reflect Hmong social values and traditional religious beliefs" (Cha 2003, 3).

An unfortunate consequence of these religious conversions has been occasional rifts between traditional and Christian Hmong. During my interviews, Christian Hmong accuse traditional Hmong of "worshipping evil," while those who practice the traditional religion allege that Christian Hmong do not separate themselves from their native beliefs as much as they like to think they do. As with many of the Hmong resettlement challenges, the conflicts between traditional religious practice and Christianity—or, more generally, United States society—appear to have affected Hmong men differently, given their role as spiritual caretakers of the family. These various resettlement issues are reflected in changes in the way night-mares have been experienced.

Dab tsog, I learned, behaves as indiscriminately as other cultures' night-mares; it is not selective about its victims and attacks both animist and Christian Hmong. Bay Lee, a thirty-five-year-old woman, told me about an attack she experienced after her conversion to Christianity. In 1988, she was living in south Stockton, an area then known for its high crime rate. It was early in the morning, still dark, and Lee and her son were the only ones home.

LEE: Right before it happened, my husband was going out. I went to bed again. I was almost asleep, but not yet. I heard that someone is coming through the door—and then right after that, someone came to me and was pressing me down. I couldn't even move and I could not open my eyes. I was very, very scared. After a while, it finally left me.

ADLER: Which way were you sleeping?

LEE: I was on my back and I felt someone was holding me down. I called my son to come and help me. I felt like I was calling, but only these sounds came out [groans]. This happened for a while and then, finally, it went away. I heard it walking out, and then I was okay. . . . After it left, I knew it was what we call *tsog tsuam,* but when I could not move, could not breathe, I was afraid—afraid someone came in—broke into the house.

ADLER: What did you try to do to make it go away?

LEE: There was nothing I could do. The spirit came to me and made me scared. At first I thought it was my husband, but then I was afraid and didn't know who it was. It was like a man in black clothes.[17] I just try to yell—try to yell real hard. If you just try to yell, try to yell, again and again, then the spirit will go away. Or, if someone is sleeping near you, you try to yell, and a sound will come out a little, and they will wake up and try to help you, and the spirit will go away.

Lee had converted to Christianity in 1980 (within two years of her arrival in the United States), but even eight years of living as a Christian did not protect her from an attack by the evil spirit she still knew as *tsog tsuam.* In describing methods of preventing the attacks, she explains: "In the old tradition, if that happens, then they need a shaman to come and give them the metal for the neck [that is, a twisted metal neck ring] or ankle, but the Christians—now I am Christian— I just pray and pray." Of the 118 people I interviewed, 115 described the attacks using traditional Hmong religious concepts, regardless of their personal religious affiliation. Only three Christian Hmong attributed the night-mare attacks exclusively to demons in the Christian sense.

The difference between *dab tsog* attacks on men and women is highlighted in the experience of Neng Kue, thirty-three, who came to the United States in 1983 after four years in a Thai refugee camp. He was only visited by *dab tsog* once, shortly after his arrival.

First, I was surprised, but right away, I got real scared. I was lying in bed. I was so tired, because I was working very hard then. I wanted to go to school, but I had no money. I kept waking up, because I was thinking so much about my problems. I heard a noise, but when I turned—tried— I could not move. My bedroom looked the same, but I could see—in the corner, a dark shape was coming to me. It came to the bed, over my feet, my legs. It was very heavy, like a heavy weight over my whole body, my legs, my chest. My chest was frozen—like I was drowning, I had no air.

I tried to yell so someone sleeping very close to me will hear. I tried to move—using a force that I can—a strength that I can have. I thought, "What can I do about this?" After a long time, it went away—it just left. I got up and turned all the lights on. I was afraid to sleep again.

Kue was twenty-five years old at the time of the nocturnal attack and living with his mother and father.

I needed a shaman. My parents are already Christian, but they are not really and truly believers—still, they don't use shamans anymore. My cousins still do it—they do it for their family. They call a shaman and do something to prevent *dab tsog* again. It is especially important for sons. They helped me.

Kue also emphasizes the importance of taking immediate action after an attack in order to prevent a recurrence: "Some people have *dab tsog* several times, and that drives you—you are really scared. You have to do something—call a shaman, make a sacrifice, change the place of your bed." Once again, it is clear that recurring attacks must be prevented, ideally by establishing the reason for the repeated visits (through a shaman's intercession) and appeasing the spirit (through a sacrifice), but at the very least by tricking the spirit. The problem of repeated attacks is exacerbated and victims' terror is intensified because, in most cases, people "don't use shamans anymore."

In an effort to learn more about Hmong interpretations of the differences between *dab tsog* attacks on Christians and animists, I asked Tong Yee Yang, a forty-year-old man who had come to the United States in 1977, whether he thought that Christian Hmong were still attacked by *dab tsog*.

YANG: Yes, they are. But they believe that somehow God will get rid of those things. They try to change their beliefs and some are devoted to their new religion. It might help [laughs]. If you have a shaman, and you do the rituals, that will help. The problem is that many Christians believe that if you strongly believe in God, the chance that *dab tsog* will disturb you will be lesser. Sure, if you strongly believe in your religion, and you say, "I will believe this until my last breath," it will help you. But many Christian Hmong don't believe this strongly. If you are in a neutral—you know, not there and not there—and you still have a doubt, chances are that *dab tsog* will be dancing around you for quite a while.

ADLER: How can you stop the attacks from happening?

YANG: A shaman has to do a ceremony. Or you can ask the priest to pray in church for that person. But you don't say, "This person has *dab tsog*, an evil spirit," you have to say, "My cousin is sick." Christians who are not Hmong do not understand. But also some Hmong—Hmong who follow the old way—do not understand.

When I asked Yang about the immediate causes of his recent night-mare attacks, he responded, "After I became Christian, it usually only happens if I don't go to church or don't pray for a long time." Yang's traditional beliefs and experiences have been incorporated into his new religion in such a way that he now interprets *dab tsog* as the outcome of his failure to meet Christian religious obligations.

The last Hmong experience I want to include is that of thirty-one-year-old Cheng Thao, a man who resettled in the United States with the aid of the Christian Missionary Alliance and subsequently converted to Christianity. He describes a night-mare attack that took place after his conversion while he was spending the night in the home of Hmong friends.

> I told them that I was visited by a devil, or *dab,* and then the wife of my friend—they are not Christian—she told me that that house had been like that for her, too. She had the same problem. She said, maybe because I was a new person in the house, the *dab tsog* came to me. I didn't know about that, but when I came into the room, I had a bad feeling there—I had a fear within myself.

Thao's use of *devil* and *dab* interchangeably reflects the ambivalence he feels about the true nature of the night-mare spirit. He is representative of a group of Christian Hmong I spoke with who appear to struggle with the absence of certain aspects of traditional Hmong religion even years after their conversion to Christianity. His fears of *tsog tsuam* are rooted in Hmong animism, ancestor worship, and shamanism, but he responds with a Christian remedy.

ADLER: Did you behave differently because you were Christian?

THAO: Oh, yes—after that happened, I prayed. I turned on the light and prayed, and then I felt better. When it happened, I tried to forget the old way. We tend to believe that God will help us, that that is nothing—nothing happened. God will help us, and we pray, and we tend to forget, and we act like nothing happened. When Hmong people become Christian they tend to forget the old beliefs and how the shamans helped, and how their ceremonies saved people's lives. They think, "Well, nothing happened like that, and now God is taking care of us." Now, when we have a bad dream or an evil spirit comes to us, we just pray and try to forget. . . . People who do not become Christian, they will worry so much, and they will have to do something—a ceremony. Christians, even though we will think sometimes, "It is an evil spirit," we will try to put it away, not think about it.

Thao's comments, in particular his observation that Christian Hmong try to forget their old traditions and beliefs, reveal the lingering influence of *dab tsog* on at least some Christian converts.

Since both Christian Hmong and traditional Hmong have died of SUNDS, an important part of my research involved learning whether Hmong of both religions experienced *dab tsog* attacks and whether they had similar responses to the events. Among the people with whom I spoke, 54 percent of traditional Hmong and 72 percent of Christian Hmong had experienced at least one night-mare. A few Christian Hmong informants described the night-mare as a demon or evil spirit in the satanic sense. Not only did Hmong of both religious groups thus experience night-mare attacks, but 98 percent of traditional Hmong and 67 percent of Christian Hmong who suggested a cause believed that these attacks resulted directly from spirits or from the absence of traditional Hmong religious practice in their lives. The psychological stress induced by night-mare attacks also affected all Hmong, irrespective of their religion. Both Christian and traditional Hmong experienced great stress regarding religious conflicts, which appeared to be heightened by night-mare attacks. In his book, *Hmong Sudden Unexpected Nocturnal Death Syndrome: A Cultural Study* (1982), Bruce Bliatout (himself Hmong) analyzes the role of religious stress in SUNDS. Bliatout suggests that, in his sample of thirty-eight Hmong (nineteen Christians and nineteen traditional Hmong) in the United States who died of SUNDS, both Christian and non-Christian Hmong were under similar stresses caused by their inability to resolve religious conflicts.

Hmong Christians could have been under stress because many probably still retained some of their traditional beliefs about ancestors and spirits, even after conversion. Those converting to Christianity often experienced peer disapproval, the anger of other clan members, and were sometimes even ostracized. Another reason conversion to Christianity may have caused increased stress levels was that many families who converted did not truly understand the concepts of Christian religion. Some of the Hmong families who resettled in Western countries converted because their sponsors were church groups or religious voluntary agencies. Out of respect for their sponsors, or desire to obtain greater services and assistance, many of these families gave up their traditional religion to become Christian without taking any comfort from their new religion. Therefore, it seems that peer pressure and lack of understanding of Christianity may cause some Hmong Christians to have anxieties about not fulfilling their expected traditional religious duties, particularly towards their ancestors. . . . The non-Christian Hmong suffered from stress over not being able to perform traditional expected religious duties. . . . Reasons for this were that, besides being fearful of the police and breaking public health laws, many complained that since they were not allowed to raise or slaughter animals in their homes, it was difficult to find adequate livestock necessary for Hmong ceremonies. Some families said that due to the disruption of village and clan groups caused by relocation, they were unable to find a Hmong religious leader or other family members to help in the performance of correct ceremonies. Others cited that living in an apartment was not conducive to providing a central pillar for ancestors to live in. (Bliatout 1982, 90–91)

I conducted a series of telephone interviews with a Hmong public health worker to learn more about the potential psychological impact of *dab tsog* on Hmong refugees in the United States. He explained that recent converts to Christianity (the group that forms the vast majority of Christian Hmong that I interviewed) are at greater risk for feelings of religious dislocation and stress from night-mare experiences than those who have practiced Christianity for many years.

MOUA: I think that, with the exception of those people whose parents already have been converted and they grew up as a Christian, they may or may not learn about all this, but they still know all the stories about *dab*. Even if you talk to Hmong Christians, they still know all these stories. . . . Those who are converted in this country, I think that they are having a more vivid experience [laughs] than those who converted back in Laos. They are, in a way—if they don't believe in it, then perhaps it is okay, but those who believe in it—I think they still are very fearful about the situation.

ADLER: Why do you think that *dab tsog* might have greater impact for those who converted to Christianity [in the United States]?

MOUA: Well, why greater impact is probably—unless they believed when they converted, and unless they believe very strongly that now either Jesus or God is going to help them, protect them. There are also many, many individuals who are converted without knowing what's going on. They just did it because their friend did it. They just did it because their sponsors are Christian. So they did it without knowing. When they converted, they continued to feel terrible. They go home and they talk to relatives and friends, and they keep saying, "Well, this is what happened to me. I already did it, but I didn't want to do it. Please continue on the old tradition," and so forth. So those individuals are the ones that, I would say, are affected the most.

Thanks to the many Hmong men and women with whom I spoke, the logic of the Hmong explanation for the role of *dab tsog* in the sudden nocturnal deaths was now clear to me.

Although it was its resonance with the night-mare that first drew me to the topic of SUNDS, part of me wished that there was no connection—that the syndrome could be attributed to causes entirely recognizable within the biomedical model and that would not, through a cultural vector, provide yet another opportunity for some to view the Hmong immigrants as exotic and alien. The traumatic recent history of the Hmong refugees (that led to their resettling in the United States) soon revealed a biocultural connection that was previously obscured by historical and geographical distance. I will now turn to this relationship to show how Hmong explanations of lethal *dab tsog* attacks can simultaneously be understood from a biomedical perspective.

6

The Night-mare and the Nocebo

Beliefs That Harm

"Human biology is comprised of neurons, neurotransmitters and synapses;
but it is also comprised of meaning, experience, knowledge and practice."

–Daniel Moerman (2002, 103)

Throughout the world, in every society, the belief exists that supernatural or magical actions can result in people's deaths. The Hmong immigrants I spoke with were, in this way, no different from people of other Eastern and Western cultures in thinking that there are nonbiological influences on health and illness. From the start of my research, I had determined to keep an open mind about the range of beliefs regarding both the night-mare and the cause(s) of SUNDS—to avoid any approach that prematurely privileged either culture or biology. So, after speaking with many Hmong men and women who shared the conviction that the nocturnal pressing spirit *dab tsog* played a role in the sudden deaths of their family members and friends, I wanted to see whether the relationship between sleep paralysis and sudden nocturnal death could be elucidated within a biomedical framework as elegantly as *dab tsog*'s influence was explained in traditional Hmong culture.

"Voodoo" Death and Psychological Stress

The classic early study of sudden death brought on by psychological stress was described in 1942 by Walter B. Cannon, head of the Department of Physiology at Harvard Medical School and a major figure in the emerging research field of psychosomatic medicine. Cannon was the first to describe the physiological mechanism responsible for the detrimental effects of "hexes" (curses) or magical rituals, the process whereby intense emotions could prove fatal. He had previously concentrated on traumatic shock, a major issue for soldiers, and was the first to describe the "fight-or-flight response" in animals (Cannon 1915).[1] Now he applied his theory of the harmful effects of the stress response to "voodoo death" in human beings; his goal was to determine "whether an ominous and persistent state of fear can end the life of a man" (1942, 176). Cannon argued that, through extreme fear (brought about by witchcraft or sorcery), the body's sympathetic nervous system is stimulated—muscles are readied for immediate action, blood vessels contract, and large amounts of adrenalin and blood sugar are produced. A less intense form of this state is a normal and healthy response to the threat of danger. "All these changes render the [organism] more efficient in physical struggle, for they supply essential conditions for continuous action of laboring muscles. Since they occur in association with the strong emotions, rage and fear, they can reasonably be interpreted as preparatory for the intense struggle which the instincts to attack or to escape may involve" (1942, 176). When the threat is not met with some action on the part of the individual, however, a state of shock may result.

> If these powerful emotions prevail, and the bodily forces are fully mobilized for action, and if this state of extreme perturbation continues in uncontrolled possession of the organism for a considerable period, without the occurrence of action, dire results may ensue. . . . The suggestion which I offer, therefore, is that "voodoo death" may be real, and that it may be explained as due to shocking emotional stress—to obvious or repressed terror. (Cannon 1942, 176)

In the situation Cannon describes—the conviction of having been cursed—the individual may be so resigned to fate that he or she refuses food and water, which only compounds the physiological problem.[2] If the condition continues, the individual is likely to die within a few days. Although Cannon's voodoo death is, therefore, not a sudden death in the sense of Hmong SUNDS, his findings regarding the physiology of emotions have had an enormous impact on the way that stress-related deaths are conceptualized.[3]

Cannon's application of the fight-or-flight theory to the study of sudden death is inspired, but he presents his argument from a disturbingly ethnocentric vantage point. He writes, "In records of anthropologists and others who have lived with primitive people in widely scattered parts of the world is the testimony that when subjected to spells or sorcery or the use of 'black magic' men may be brought to death. . . . The phenomenon is so extraordinary and so foreign to the experience of civilized people that it seems incredible" (Cannon 1942, 169). Cannon's bias is evident throughout his article: "The phenomenon is characteristically noted among aborigines—among human beings so primitive, so superstitious, so ignorant, that they feel themselves bewildered strangers in a hostile world. Instead of knowledge, they have fertile and unrestricted imaginations which fill their environment with all manners of evil spirits capable of affecting their lives disastrously" (Cannon 1942, 175). Subsequent research has shown that, on the contrary, the negative effects of emotional and psychological stress can be physiologically devastating to individuals, regardless of culture or religion. Over the ensuing half century of research, both the mechanism of voodoo death and its very existence in non-Western societies have remained subjects of extensive debate. While some researchers (e.g., Eastwell 1982) continue to maintain that voodoo death is possible, albeit with psychological factors secondary to physiological ones, others suggest that voodoo death is simply a fabrication of European and American scholars that has too hastily been accepted as evidence-based truth (Lewis 1987; Reid and Williams 1984).

Anthropologist Otniel Dror explains that, after World War II, there was a radical shift from earlier attempts to distinguish between and distance Western and "primitive" to the realization that phenomena similar to voodoo death were ubiquitous in modern experience. "Instead of relegating voodoo death to the exotic, [postwar authors] universalized voodoo death, ultimately transforming it into one of the distinct characteristics of modern life—sudden death resulting from the acute stress of modernization (Dror 2004, 76). Voodoo death was no longer considered a phenomenon exclusively associated with exotic "others." In 1957, psychobiologist Curt P. Richter suggested an alternative explanation for the trigger of sudden death. Instead of Cannon's concept of an overstimulated sympathetic nervous system, Richter posited that excessive activity of the parasympathetic nervous system was to blame. Basing his ideas on experiments with wild rats, Richter suggested that a sense of hopelessness—being trapped in a situation from which, it is perceived, there is no escape—is enough to cause death (Richter 1957). Psychiatrist George L. Engel[4] summarizes the range of psychological factors implicated in sudden deaths due to emotional stress: "Common to all is that they involve events impossible for the victims to ignore and to which their response is overwhelming excitation or giving up, or both" (Engel 1971, 771). He proposes that this combination of emotions can result in deadly outcomes, particularly in individuals with preexisting cardiovascular disease. Responding to criticism from medical researchers who ridiculed the investigation of the effects of emotional stress on health, and anticipating future studies of SUNDS, Engel observes, "Only by . . . careful scrutiny does it become possible to establish what part of folklore is fantasy and what part is fact. Certainly the use of 'folklore' or 'old wives' tales' as pejorative labels, as some skeptics are wont to do, is hardly compatible with the scientific attitude requisite for the study of natural phenomena involving life and death" (1974, 781).[5]

In increasing numbers, investigators began heeding Engel's advice, paying greater attention to social stressors and the resulting psychological and physical responses (Mishler et al. 1981). For example, oncologist Gerald W. Milton, who treated patients in an Australian melanoma clinic, became convinced of "the similarity between the westernized man dying through fear of a disease from which there is no escape and the aborigine who dies from an all-powerful spell" (1973, 1436). Milton found that, for some of his cancer patients, "the realization of impending death is a blow so terrible that they are quite unable to adjust to it, and they die rapidly before the malignancy seems to have developed enough to cause death" (1435). In a related example, in 1974, Tennessee physician Clifton Meador treated a patient for cancer of the esophagus, a disease that was considered fatal at the time. The patient died a few weeks later, but the subsequent autopsy revealed that his esophagus was perfectly healthy. He did have a few small tumors in his liver and one in his lung, but there was no evidence of life-threatening disease. Meador, interviewed three decades later, explained, "He died with cancer, but not from cancer. . . . I thought he had cancer. He thought he had cancer. Everybody around him thought he had cancer" (Holder 2007).[6]

Of particular relevance to the study of Hmong SUNDS, there is a relatively long tradition of looking to the effects of psychological stress as a factor in sudden cardiac death. Bernard Lown and colleagues sought, for example, to determine whether neurophysiologic activity can have such a profound effect on cardiac electrical properties that it can cause fibrillation (rapid, irregular contractions of the heart's muscle fibers) in the absence of cardiovascular disease. Researchers conducted a series of sleep studies during which they noted a substantial increase in irregular heartbeats during REM sleep (Lown et al. 1976). They conclude that "psychologic and neurophysiologic factors may predispose to life threatening cardiac arrhythmia in the absence of organic heart disease" (623). In another article, Lown explains that "psychologic stresses, even of brief duration, profoundly reduce the threshold for ventricular fibrillation and result in major ventricular rhythm disorders" (Lown and Verrier 1976, 1170).

Psychiatrist Peter Reich and his research group at the Brigham and Women's Hospital in Boston investigated the prevalence of acute psychological disturbances during the twenty-four hours preceding life-threatening ventricular arrhythmias.

> Malignant ventricular arrhythmias appeared to be caused by a combination of three factors: myocardial electrical instability, a stressful psychological state that burdens everyday life, and a proximate intense psychologic event. Experimental reports indicate that neural and psychological factors may affect ventricular electrical stability and provoke malignant ventricular arrhythmias through sympathetic arousal. . . . This suggests that emotional disturbances may play a role in the pathogenesis of arrhythmias in a limited but notable number of patients. (Reich et al. 1981, 235)

Cardiologist Michael A. Brodsky and colleagues focused on patients with life-threatening rapid, irregular heartbeats (tachyarrhythmia) who also experience marked psychological stress. The researchers suggest that their findings may give insight into the "syndrome of sudden death in Asian immigrants," and they conclude that "psychological stress can be an important factor in the development of life-threatening ventricular tachyarrhythmia. This may be particularly important in individuals without detectable heart disease" (Brodsky et al. 1987,

2067). Toward the end of the twentieth century, scientific interest in and acceptance of the impact of emotional stress on cardiac health thus increased. Could the Hmong sudden deaths, like *dab tsog* itself, also be understood as the interaction of biological and cultural influences on health?

In 1984, a group of physicians published the case histories of three Southeast Asian men who had been successfully resuscitated after sudden nocturnal cardiac arrest (Otto et al. 1984). On the basis of cardiographic studies of the three men during their hospitalization, ventricular arrhythmias were the primary events underlying the cardiac arrests. The cause of the arrhythmias was unknown, but the event that most likely precedes SUNDS deaths was demonstrated. After analyzing eighteen hearts obtained through autopsies of SUNDS victims, Robert Kirschner and colleagues concluded that conduction system anomalies may be the substrate for sleep-related cardiac arrhythmias and sudden death. The investigators noted that the syndrome's underlying condition was, for the most part, "clinically silent" and that fatal or near fatal episodes probably result from rare disturbances in cardiac electrical conduction (Kirschner, Eckner, and Baron 1986).

The following year, Roy Gibson Parrish, of the Centers for Disease Control, summarized the results of SUNDS studies, including the CDC surveillance, and suggested a possible mechanism for the deaths.

> SUNDS victims appear to have abnormalities, possibly hereditary, of the tissues that conduct electrical impulses through the heart and are responsible for its orderly beating. Under most ordinary circumstances these abnormalities produce no significant clinical problems, and the affected individuals are unaware that they may be in danger. Only in times of unusual stress and possibly in conjunction with other, as yet undefined factors are these people at risk of developing abnormal electrical impulses in the heart that result in ventricular fibrillation and sudden death. (Parrish 1988, 290)

Although the existence of these underlying cardiac conduction system abnormalities contributed to the understanding of the potential mechanism of SUNDS, the anomalies alone provide no explanation for the purported absence of the sudden deaths in Laos, the preponderance of deaths during the first two years after the Hmong immigrants' arrival in the United States, or the fact that a clinically silent problem would suddenly manifest so violently as to cause death.

Placebo's Evil Twin

Unlike the placebo, the nocebo phenomenon produces an unpleasant or harmful outcome as a consequence of a person's beliefs. Nocebo effects are not uncommon in clinical practice. In "white coat hypertension," patients have elevated blood pressure at the doctor's office, but not in other settings (most likely due to stress, fear, and pessimism experienced during the clinic visit) (Verdecchia et al. 2002). Nausea and vomiting are common side effects that occur after chemotherapy—but around 60 percent of patients undergoing chemotherapy start feeling sick before their treatment. This "anticipatory nausea" is at least partly due to negative expectation (Morrow and Dobkin 1988). The nocebo effect can also be seen in the ongoing Framingham Heart Study, which was begun in 1948 to identify common factors that contribute to cardiovascular disease by following its development over time in participants without any overt symptoms. Women who believed they were prone to heart disease were found to be nearly four times as likely to die as women with similar risk factors (e.g., high blood pressure, excessive weight, high cholesterol) who did not believe they were particularly susceptible (Eaker, Pinsky, and Castelli 1992).

The effect of the nocebo is more poorly understood and more rarely taken into account than the widely known placebo, most likely because of ethical considerations. In many situations, it is not acceptable to induce negative expectations that may lead to an actual worsening of symptoms. In one early study, though, people with asthma were given an innocuous saline solution to inhale but were told that the substance contained irritants that might temporarily worsen their condition. The group experienced increased airway resistance and a corresponding perception of increased breathing difficulties. When the same substance was administered again, but this time described as therapeutic, airway resistance decreased and easy breathing returned (Luparello et al. 1968). In a follow-up, double-blind experiment, the researchers randomized people with asthma to four study arms: two groups were given a bronchodilator, and the other two were given a bronchoconstrictor. Half the people in each group were told that they were being given a bronchodilator, and the other half were told that they were given a bronchoconstrictor. For each substance administered, misinformation about the substance reduced its physiological effectiveness by almost 50 percent (Luparello et al. 1970).

A more recent example of the nocebo effect is found in a study designed to explore the frequently reported symptom of headaches in connection with mobile phone use. The researchers designed a double-blind provocation study to determine whether exposure to radio frequency fields from mobile phones results in more head pain or discomfort than sham exposure. People who regularly experience head pain or discomfort during or shortly after mobile phone calls were recruited to participate. The exposure system consisted of one radio-frequency antenna and one sham exposure antenna mounted symmetrically outside a box on either side of the subject's head. Participants were informed that they would sometimes be exposed to fields from a mobile phone and sometimes not—they were not told which one of the antennae was used. After analyzing participants' descriptions of symptoms, the researchers concluded that "exposure to radio frequency fields from mobile phones does not cause pain or discomfort in the head or other symptoms, even in individuals carefully selected according to the criterion of a specific sensitivity to mobile phone use. In the majority of pairs of radio frequency and sham exposures, sham resulted in the most severe symptoms. The most likely explanation for our results is that the symptoms are due to negative expectations, i.e. a nocebo effect" (Oftedal et al. 2007, 454).

In a related cross-sectional study of Scandinavian mobile phone users, scientists found a correlation between call duration and prevalence of symptoms (Sandstrom et al. 2001). In contrast, however, a similar study among students in Iran did not reveal any association between symptom severity and the use of mobile phones (Mortazavi, Ahmadi, and Shariati 2007). Neurologist Lars Jacob Stovner and colleagues believe that the discrepancy in symptoms between the two study populations can be traced to the differing societal contexts of the participants. They suggest that the lack of mass media interest in the potential health risk of mobile phone radiation in Iran may explain this negative finding. In Norway, however, "the former prime minister and ex-president of the World Health Organization has received and still receives widespread media coverage of her contention that she gets headache from mobile phone use" (Stovner et al. 2008, 70). Because expectations are largely learned from the cultural environment, nocebo effects are thus likely to vary from place to place (Hahn 1997).

Of particular relevance to the study of the nocebo and Hmong SUNDS are the pathogenic effects of ethnomedicine, the medical beliefs and practices of a culture. "Ethnomedicogenic" illness and healing is a concept based on the premise that, in any given society, an individual's beliefs play a significant role in both disease production and healing (Hahn and Kleinman 1983). The two extremes of ethnomedicogenic phenomena, from placebo and faith healing on the therapeutic side to voodoo death and sudden death on the pathogenic side, can be thought of as ends of a continuum. These health/illness events are based on an "interaction between culture and physiology mediated by central nervous system processing of symbolic perception in experience" (Hahn and Kleinman 1983, 16). The nocebo phenomenon is essentially a side effect of human culture.

> A society's ethnomedicine constructs medical reality in that it informs both patient and practitioner about how symptoms and conditions are distinguished, what courses they run in syndromes and why, how these conditions may be ameliorated, and how symptoms and their dynamics fit in a larger order of agency, power, and value. An ethnomedicine is an element also in the production of that medical reality, by the organization of medical facets of social life from the first recognition of symptoms to healing. The wider culture, of which ethnomedicine is a part, also profoundly affects the organization of disease and healing in society. (Hahn and Kleinman 1983, 16–17)

The categories of ethnomedicine—including biomedicine, one of American society's ethnomedicines—not only describe conditions of sickness, but also foster those conditions by establishing beliefs that they may occur. "Expectations are a bridge connecting our culture and our bodies" (Hahn 1995, 90). Anthropologist Daniel Moerman has broadened the understanding of the effects of the nocebo (and placebo) to include situations in which an individual has no conscious expectation. Preferring the term "meaning effect," Moerman asserts that "people know things, and experience them meaningfully. They respond to what things mean (whether they 'expect' it or not)" (Moerman 2002, 126). The nocebo thus represents the transformation of meaning and belief into undesired physiological processes. Importantly, this type of mind-body connection is compatible with the traditional Hmong worldview regarding health and illness. Michael A. Ingall, a psychiatrist at Brown University who has worked with Hmong men and women in Rhode Island, explains that most of these immigrants "readily accept the concept of psychosomatic illness, which is seen as a manifestation of the relationship between the body and spirit. When the body is not well, the spirit becomes troubled. Conversely, if the spirit is not at ease, the body develops disease" (Ingall 1984, 369). The idea of *dab tsog* harming sleepers through a connection between mind and body is plausible according to traditional Hmong belief. In order to complete this conceptualization within the biomedical paradigm, however, it is necessary to fit one last piece of the puzzle: Is there a biological narrative for *dab tsog*'s final, lethal act?

Unmasking the Brugada Syndrome

In 1986, Pedro Brugada, a cardiologist who specializes in cardiac arrhythmias, examined the ECG (electrocardiogram) of one of his patients and noticed a strange pattern that he had never seen before—an unusual shape that was reminiscent of a shark's fin. Over the next few years, he searched for this electrical pattern in other victims of cardiac arrest, but it was not until 1992, after he had collected seven more of these unusual ECGs, that Brugada (together with his brother, Josep), published findings regarding the "recurrent episodes of aborted sudden death unexplainable by currently known diseases" (Brugada and Brugada 1992, 1391). The deaths had common clinical and electrocardiographic features that indicated they were part of a distinct and new clinical entity—later named the Brugada syndrome.

Brugada syndrome is a rare, inherited condition that causes a disruption of the heart's normal rhythm. The disorder, which appears to be eight to ten times more common in men,[7] can lead to uncoordinated electrical activity in the heart's lower chambers (ventricles), an abnormality that is known as ventricular arrhythmia. If untreated, the irregular heartbeats can cause syncope (fainting), seizures, difficulty breathing, or sudden death. These complications most commonly occur at night, when the affected person is asleep (Matsuo et al.

1999). SUNDS is found in Southeast Asia (particularly Thailand and Cambodia), Japan, and the Philippines, and it causes sudden cardiac death during nighttime sleep, usually in men. Based on clinical and epidemiological research, scientists now believe that SUNDS and Brugada syndrome are the same disorder.

In Brugada syndrome, the heart typically has a normal structure, but an ECG can reveal impaired electrical activity. Although the disorder is associated with a peculiar ECG pattern, the characteristic ECG changes are not consistently present in many patients. Symptoms often appear with no warning, and a seemingly healthy person may suffer sudden cardiac arrest from an arrhythmia. There is presently no cure for Brugada syndrome. The best therapy for people who are clinically found to be at high risk for the disorder is an implantable cardioverter-defibrillator. (Sewn under the skin of the upper chest with wires passing through veins directly into the heart, defibrillators are programmed to detect cardiac arrhythmia and correct it by delivering an electrical shock.)

Scientists have found mutations in the genes that are known to influence the electrical activity of the heart. Gene SCN5A, for example, controls the flow of sodium ions into heart cells. A mutation in this gene is responsible for the deadly arrhythmias in the Brugada syndrome.[8] However, only 15 to 30 percent of patients diagnosed with Brugada syndrome have mutations in the SCN5A gene (Miura, Nakamura, and Ohe 2008). In affected people without an identified genetic mutation, the cause of Brugada syndrome is often unknown. Cardiologist Barry London, lead author on a study identifying another gene (GPD1L) whose mutation appears to be linked to Brugada syndrome (London et al. 2007), articulates a significant point: "Patients with Brugada syndrome only rarely have symptoms; they have this genetic mutation all the time. So, the question now is, why do arrhythmias or sudden death happen on any one particular day? Something else is happening concurrently with this mutation to trigger the potentially lethal rhythm problems" (ScienceDaily 2007).

The true prevalence of Brugada syndrome in the general population is unknown and difficult to estimate because diagnostic features may be subtle, concealed, or transient. Researchers have investigated a number of events that might "unmask" the hidden or silent disorder (i.e., force it to manifest clinically). There are a variety of pharmacologic drug challenges that can be used in cases of suspected Brugada syndrome to trigger the characteristic ECG features and thereby identify patients at risk of sudden death (Wichter et al. 2006). There also appear to be naturally occurring events that predispose people to Brugada syndrome. Assessments of heart rate variability reveal impaired autonomic function at night, which could predispose to the occurrence of ventricular fibrillation (Krittayaphong et al. 2003) and "intermittent fluctuations in cardiac sympathetic and parasympathetic tone during REM sleep might trigger ventricular arrhythmias, increasing vulnerability to sleep related ventricular tachycardia and sudden cardiac death" (Garcia-Touchard et al. 2007, 288).

Autonomic instability during REM sleep could be significant if the same type of flux is present in sleep-onset REM.

Scientists continue to develop noninvasive diagnostic tools to unmask Brugada syndrome. In a study that recalls Scrooge's attempt to blame his vision of Marley's ghost on overindulging in a late-night repast in Charles Dickens's *A Christmas Carol*,[9] Takanori Ikeda and colleagues at the Kyorin University School of Medicine in Japan explored food intake as a modulator. Participants were urged to eat a large meal within twenty minutes—the food consisted of "dishes preferred by the subject such as hamburgers, pizza, noodles, rice balls, sushi, or tempura" (Ikeda et al. 2006, 603). The investigators studied changes in ECGs before and after patients hastily consumed their generously sized feast, and they concluded that a stomach rapidly filled with a large meal is associated with ECG abnormalities. In other words, a large meal consumed before sleep may be one of the factors contributing to the occurrence of ventricular fibrillation in patients with Brugada syndrome. Can *dab tsog* unmask Brugada syndrome, as well?

Night-mare and Sudden Death in Other Cultures

Neither the night-mare nor SUNDS/Brugada syndrome is specific to the Hmong. The night-mare is, in fact, traditionally associated with sudden nocturnal deaths in other Asian cultures. How is it, then, that a traditional Hmong spirit can be involved in SUNDS? In all of the settings in which the sudden nocturnal deaths occur—including Japan, where the disorder is called *pokkuri* ("sudden unexplained death at night"), Thailand (*lai-tai,* "dying during sleep"), and the Philippines (*bangungut,* "moaning and dying during sleep")—there exist traditions of night-mare attacks that can be lethal. Although the Hmong refugee and immigrant experiences are my focus, it is important to note that some people from other Southeast Asian groups also attribute SUNDS deaths to night-mare attacks.

We have seen that neither the night-mare nor Brugada syndrome is a culture-bound syndrome; they are not disorders specific to one society or cultural setting. A detailed discussion of potentially parallel phenomena is beyond my present aim, but a quick look at cultural understandings of Khmu and Thai sudden deaths illustrates that at least some people from both of these groups perceive a connection between night-mare spirit attacks and sudden deaths in situations of extreme psychological stress. Like the Hmong, the Khmu are a highland Lao people who were recruited by the U.S. Central Intelligence Agency to fight as guerrillas against the Pathet Lao. They, too, fled to Thailand in 1975, and approximately 3,000 Khmu eventually resettled in the United States. I spoke with one Khmu man, Chantha Santikhara, who directed a mutual assistance association in central California. His male cousin (who practiced the traditional Khmu religion) and his nephew (Christian) both died of SUNDS. Santikhara's relatives attribute both deaths to evil spirits.

Before discussing SUNDS, which the Khmu call *sih han* ("sleep and die"), I ask the generic question about sleep paralysis features. In reply, he describes the Khmu night-mare spirit, which he refers to as *hrooy keut*. According to Santikhara, who converted to Christianity in Thailand, *hrooy keut* can kill either by suffocating its victim or by enticing the victim's spirit away from its body. He describes all the classic elements of the traditional night-mare attack, including the feature of lying in a supine position. "*Hrooy keut* comes to people sleeping on their back. Parents, grandparents warned us not to sleep lying on the back." He goes on to explain that people are particularly susceptible to *hrooy keut* attacks when they are sleeping in the jungle.

> For this reason, when Khmu go hunting, especially the water buffalo—the bigger the animal, the more bad spirits you have to be careful of—there are stories about people who go hunting the big animals and then go to sleep at night. Everyone who goes to that one place to hunt, they always die. Nobody comes back. But two people went and tried a new way. They both slept in a line, with their feet touching—not side by side. And then when the spirit came, it tried to sit on one guy, but it looked like the other guy was going to come [laughs] and grab the spirit. So the spirit couldn't do anything and had to go. That's why they say, "When you go to the forest, try to sleep that way."

Santikhara explains that a visit from *hrooy keut* is "frightening" because of the fear of suffocation. In reference to his own encounter with a night-mare, he reveals, "I'm scared, too—even though I don't believe in spirits." Although the capacity of traditional Khmu spirits to kill human beings is not a part of Santikhara's personal Christian worldview, he speculates that people who die of SUNDS have become so weakened emotionally and psychologically that what they perceive to be a *hrooy keut* attack can actually kill them.

Men in northeast Thailand perceive a link between the local night-mare and *lai tai*. In an effort to prevent sudden nocturnal deaths, some men have taken steps that may seem odd to those unfamiliar with night-mare manifestations such as the succubus. Blaming female night-mare spirits for sexually attacking and then killing their victims, surviving men endeavor to fool the spirits into thinking they are women. If several young men die in a village within a short time, the survivors employ a variety of strategies to protect themselves, including wearing nail polish or women's clothing to bed and setting up large wooden phalluses around the house (Hinton and Good 2009; Johnson 1991). Because of the unexplained nocturnal deaths and the beliefs regarding their cause, northeastern Thai men greatly fear sensations of shortness of breath upon awakening. If this fear reaches unreasonable levels, people refer to it as "fear-of-sudden-unexplained-nocturnal-death illness" (*rook klua lai tai*). In this case, "the biology of panic, gender construction, biological gender differences, and culturally generated fears are in dynamic interaction" (Hinton and Good 2009, 199). In light of the robust traditions of established links between local night-mare spirits and *sih han* and *lai tai* (as well as *pokkuri* and *bangungut*), there appears to be a culturally mediated association. Within the biomedical paradigm, this connection can be understood as (a) primarily biological with cultural elaboration or (b) a cultural tradition that has the power to cause illness (and perhaps death) in (genetically) susceptible individuals.

Another example of psychological stress and night-mare as factors in the sudden deaths of a non-Hmong group is found in Thai construction workers in Singapore, Saudi Arabia, Iraq, Kuwait, and Brunei. Michael Brodsky, the arrhythmia specialist, believes that SUNDS deaths are stress-related. He found that Thai workers who died in their sleep were laboring seven days a week, 12 hours per day, for meager wages: "They were treated like indentured servants, almost like slaves. . . . If you put people in hopeless situations, in strange lands, there's no doubt they can lose the will to live" (Brody 1990, 12).

Manifold Meanings and Local Biologies

Returning to SUNDS, we have seen that, even in the context of widely shared concepts of biomedicine and scientific sleep research, experiences of sleep paralysis vary significantly and hold different meanings for different people. The nightmare is polysemic—it can mean different things at different times and in different contexts.[10] The same sensations that herald (or create) terror in one cultural model may have a positive value (for example, an inspiring out-of-body experience) in another. Sleep laboratories can only record the neurophysiological correlates of the night-mare; for its actual meaning, we must depend on the narratives of the experiencers, narratives that are heavily influenced by cultural beliefs. Biomedicine characteristically separates "disease," an objectively verified disorder, from "illness," a patient's subjective experience. It was this oversimplified dichotomy that prompted George Engel to theorize a "biopsychosocial model" in order to consider all factors that play a role in health and sickness. A mind-body approach, similarly, requires a biocultural model, which situates illness at the interface of biology and culture (Morris 2000). In order to comprehend night-mare/sleep paralysis and SUNDS/Brugada syndrome, we must take into account both biology and culture; an attempt to understand these disorders of the body, separate from their cultural dimensions, is incomplete.

The seemingly universal pattern of human physiology makes us forget that there is tremendous variation in the ways that people experience and understand their own bodies, health, and illness.

> In so far as a culture (German, Navajo, Zulu) is a skein of meanings, understandings, beliefs, and knowledge, stitched together somehow by

metaphors, institutions, and memories, and in so far as these things can affect individual lives, it seems reasonable to anticipate that these factors will work themselves out differently in different places in the world. . . . The same item . . . can be expected to mean different things in different places, and, therefore, it can be expected to have different effects there. (Moerman 2002, 84)

The role of the night-mare in SUNDS exemplifies Moerman's idea of the "meaning response": since meaning has biological consequences, and meanings vary across cultures, biology can operate differently in different contexts. In other words, biology is "local"—the "same" biological processes in different places have different "effects" on people.[11]

"Sleep Debt" and Chronic Stress

We know that a sufficient quantity of REM sleep is essential for healthy, normal sleep. The homeostatic regulation of REM sleep is expressed by progressively more frequent attempts to enter REM and by a compensatory rebound after the deprivation ends. Significantly, the deprivation of REM sleep also generates REM sleep at sleep onset in healthy sleepers (Hishikawa 1976; Kryger, Roth, and Dement 2000; Rechtschaffen and Dement 1969). People deprived of REM sleep have a greater chance of experiencing sleep-onset REM, which can manifest as sleep paralysis and hypnic hallucinations—in other words, night-mares.

There are indications that Hmong night-mare sufferers and SUNDS victims had experienced disrupted and insufficient sleep. Lemoine and Mougne observed that "there was often evidence that the victims had been exhausted, combining full-time jobs with demanding night school classes or other enterprises. In quite a few cases the fatal sleep had occurred immediately after a family row or late TV watching or interrupted sleep" (1983, 18). Tragically, some Hmong men, fearing that deep sleep could bring about their deaths, set their alarm clocks to awaken them every twenty or thirty minutes (Holtan et al. 1984), or they used other strategies, such as a loud television, radio noise, or bright lights in the bedroom at night. This type of sleep disruption may have actually caused sleep-onset REM and night-mares.

When the number of SUNDS deaths peaked in 1981, its rapid rate of increase created much interest among biomedical researchers. Since that time, the number of deaths and the crude death rate among Hmong men has fallen steadily (apart from a slight increase in 1988). This pattern appears to be associated with the stress of relocation to the United States, since the number of deaths among Laotian refugees in the United States rose and fell in association with the amount of time that the men had been in the United States.[12] A 1988 update on SUNDS cases reported that the "median length of time in the United States for the 88 of the 117 decedents for whom time in the United States was known was 17 months," and it linked the decline in the number of deaths with decreased numbers of incoming Southeast Asian refugees. "The decline in [SUNDS] cases may be related to this decline in newly arrived Southeast Asian refugees, since most deaths occur within the first two years after arrival in the United States" (Centers for Disease Control 1988, 569).

The types of stress that the Hmong men and women described would be expected to manifest most strongly during the initial arrival period, which is characterized by the greatest change but, often, the least amount of available emotional support. Conversely, a reason for the decline in the number, followed by the cessation, of deaths appears to be the fact that later Hmong arrivals had many more forms of support available (e.g., close-knit communities, restored clan ties, greater possibility for traditional religious practice). The 1987 report from the Centers for Disease Control strengthens these speculations:

> The decline in both the number of cases and the crude incidence sug-
> gests that some risk factor present soon after the refugees arrive in the
> United States may be important and that this risk factor diminishes with
> time. . . . Although this pattern is less compatible with a congenital car-
> diac abnormality or a sleep disturbance, hypotheses concerning these two
> risk factors may still be viable if most susceptibles have died or if some
> environmental factor (such as stress) in combination with the cardiac
> abnormality or sleep disturbance is causative. (Parrish et al. 1987, 53)

If sudden cardiac death can be precipitated by the psychological stress of a *dab tsog* attack, why was it not induced by one of the series of pre-resettlement traumas that the Hmong had sustained? The village raids in Laos and the crossing of the Mekong River are just two examples of traumatic situations that one might expect to be sufficiently stressful to cause this type of cardiac arrhythmia. From the biomedical perspective, however, these deaths are not due to psychological stress in isolation, but to the effect of psychological stress on a person susceptible to Brugada syndrome. It is my contention that in the context of severe and ongoing stress related to cultural disruption and national resettlement (exacerbated by intense feelings of powerlessness about existence in the United States), and from the perspective of a belief system in which evil spirits have the power to kill men who do not fulfill their religious obligations, the solitary Hmong man confronted by the numinous terror of the night-mare (and aware of its murderous intent) can die of SUNDS.

Dab Tsog and Sudden Deaths: From Laos to the United States

Experiences and expectations of *dab tsog* attacks in the native Hmong context of highland Laos differed from those of the new Hmong environment in the United

States. In Laos, there was collective support for people who suffered from night-mare attacks, including broad exposure to narratives (legends and memorates) detailing experiences of other people, opportunities to recount one's own experiences to shamans and clan leaders, and access to community rituals to prevent the unwanted incident from occurring or, failing that, to remedy an existing situation. The traditional means of preventing *dab tsog* attacks included performing shamanic and familial rituals to ensure the safety and contentment of one's souls, caring for tame spirits (especially the ancestor spirits) through "feeding" and a variety of other rituals, and avoiding wild spirits (nature spirits and untamed evil spirits) and their territory. Remedies against future attacks involved the services of a shaman as diagnostician and, frequently, intervener (fighter, bargainer) on behalf of the *dab tsog*'s victim in the spirit world. This elaborate system for dealing with night-mares, however, did not alter the fact that *dab tsog* attacks experienced by individuals in Laos were terrifying. Nevertheless, as I have related, none of the Hmong men and women I interviewed was aware of sudden nocturnal deaths occurring in Laos. As one person explained, because of traditional countermeasures taken in Laos, SUNDS deaths did not occur prior to the Hmong exodus. "There were night-mares, but the sudden death was unheard of. It might have happened, but I never heard of it." In Laos, night-mare attacks occurred in a cultural setting that was equipped to deal with them; victims of *dab tsog* had collective assistance in terms of experience and explanatory models of traditional Hmong culture.

In the United States, traditional support was disrupted by the tremendous social transformation that the early Hmong immigrants underwent in terms of hasty conversions to Christianity, the inability to practice traditional rituals, the dispersal of tightly knit clans, the breakdown of the traditional age and gender hierarchy, and the need to learn a new language and to procure new means of employment. Hmong men suffered disproportionately from serious emotional stress due to changes in the traditional gender and generational hierarchy and the sudden inability to lead and provide for their families both financially and spiritually.

Traditional Hmong men faced great difficulty in practicing their religion as they had done in Laos.[13] The inability to obtain animals for sacrifice, the disruption of clan ties, and the scarcity of shamans all contributed to the problem of performing expected religious duties. Many Christian Hmong men also retained traditional beliefs and had anxieties about not fulfilling their religious requirements. Some Christian Hmong converted out of a sense of obligation to church sponsors, and many experienced peer disapproval and clan ostracization. Although the more devout Christians with whom I spoke denied any ambivalence, many of the Christian Hmong participants described ways in which they combined the two religions in order to prevent incurring the wrath of Hmong spirits. It is striking that, of the Christian Hmong who offered an explanation for the cause of the sudden nocturnal deaths, 74 percent suggested an etiology that was directly spirit-related or involved the absence of traditional religion and ritual from their lives.

In addition to the conflict between Hmong traditional religion and Christianity, the early immigrants experienced a host of hardships including language and employment problems, changing generational and gender roles, survivor guilt, and trauma-induced emotional and psychological disorders. These changes can affect all immigrants to varying degrees, but Hmong men, in particular, experienced a dramatic alteration in their social roles. This gender dichotomy is mirrored by the discrepancy in the sudden nocturnal deaths. Since both Hmong men and women suffered from night-mare attacks, it was essential to learn people's views regarding the reason the deaths occurred overwhelmingly among men. The answer lies in the meaning of night-mare attacks in traditional Hmong culture. Both Hmong men and women explained that, in addition to other religious requirements, one's ancestor spirits must be fed annually. If the ancestor spirits were neglected, they became angry and deserted the individual—the head-of-household—leaving him vulnerable to evil spirit attacks. A direct causal relationship was seen between the failure to perform traditional Hmong rituals and *dab tsog* attacks. (Etiologies related to either traditional spirits or to the lack of traditional religious practice constituted 81 percent of the nightmare causes suggested overall.) The inability to fulfill roles and responsibilities with regard to religion (as well as in their lives generally) was perceived to have a calamitous impact on the well being of Hmong men. Although Hmong women did experience night-mare attacks and were aware of the roles of both spirits and the absence of traditional religious practices in the sudden nocturnal deaths, they also knew that *dab tsog* would seek out their husbands, fathers, or brothers as the individuals held accountable. As one Hmong woman recalled of her own nightmare experience: "Even though I was very, very scared, I thought it was good my husband wasn't there, so the spirit wouldn't hurt him."

Traditional Hmong culture has sustained a severe disruption. The Hmong people have undergone a seemingly endless series of traumatic experiences: the war in Laos; the Pathet Lao takeover and subsequent Hmong persecution (including the threat of genocide); the harrowing nighttime escapes through jungles and across the Mekong River; the hardships of refugee camps in Thailand; and, finally, resettlement in the United States, with not only housing, income, language, and employment concerns, but also the separation of families and clans, inability to practice traditional religion, and hasty conversions to Christianity. When *dab tsog* tormented sleepers in Laos, it did so in a sociocultural context that sustained a fundamental structure of support. Hmong shamans conducted prescribed rituals designed to ascertain the nature of the individual's transgression and sought to appease the angry spirits in order to prevent the possibility of the sleeper's death during a subsequent nocturnal encounter. In the United States, though the majority of Hmong retained many of their traditional beliefs, they had lost their religious leaders and ritual responses. The insular communities that characterized Hmong life in Laos appear to have fostered traditional cultural practices whose presence alleviated, but whose subsequent loss provoked, feelings of terror and impending death associated with negative spirit encounters. Therefore, although the *dab tsog* attacks in Laos were akin to the worldwide night-mare tradition, they were transformed by the peculiar stresses of the Hmong refugee experience. The power of traditional belief in *dab tsog*—compounded by such factors as the trauma of war, migration, rapid acculturation, and the inability to practice traditional healing and ritual—can cause cataclysmic psychological stress.[14]

Many of the Hmong with whom I spoke proposed that their traditional nightmare spirit is the culprit in the sudden nocturnal deaths that occurred in the 1980s and early 1990s. Can this traditional explanation also be understood meaningfully outside of Hmong culture? The answer is *yes*. Sleep paralysis is certainly not fatal; however, under certain conditions, *dab tsog* can kill. There are, in the end, more than two explanations for the Hmong sudden deaths. The traditional Hmong understanding of the lethal *dab tsog* attack and the biomedical account of a rare, inherited cardiac arrhythmia are complementary alternatives. For me, though, the most complete view includes local variations in both culture and biology. A biocultural perspective on the phenomenon sees the interplay between biology (a genetic cardiac conduction disorder) and meaning (*dab tsog* as a trigger for cataclysmic psychological stress) at the heart of the Hmong sudden nocturnal deaths. The Brugada syndrome consists of genetic abnormalities of the heart that remain silent or hidden until a stressor, such as *dab tsog,* supervenes and triggers a cascade of physiological and pathologic responses, ending in sudden death.

In 2005, the closing of the last Thai refugee camps prompted the largest influx of Hmong refugees to the United States since the 1980s—the time of the peak incidence in SUNDS deaths. With more than five thousand Hmong refugees resettling in the Twin Cities, some physicians wondered whether SUNDS would resurface. When Neal Holtan, the Minneapolis doctor who became an international expert on SUNDS, was asked whether SUNDS might reappear among the new immigrants, he answered, "I think it will" (Meier 2004). Bruce Bliatout also worried that stresses will increase for new Hmong residents arriving from Thailand: "They've been living in refugee camps for almost 30 years, they have no work, they haven't seen the world. They don't know the language, how to drive, how to look for a job. Relatives and social-services agencies will do their best to help them settle. Hopefully this will eliminate SUNDS. But I don't know" (Meier 2004). For many others in the Hmong community, though, the fear of SUNDS is now over. Xuoa Thao, a St. Paul family medicine physician who sees mostly Hmong patients, explains, "I've been here nine years and have yet to see one case. Nobody even talks about it anymore" (Meier 2004).

Conclusion

Sixty years ago, only a small number of scientists and health-care practitioners were aware of sleep paralysis, although millions of Americans were experiencing the phenomenon. Even when sleep researchers began to learn about the neurophysiology of sleep paralysis, the impact of the personal experience remained obscure. Today, despite the high prevalence of (and growing interest in) sleep paralysis in the United States, the experience is only rarely recounted. This is partly due to the fact that public awareness of the night-mare is a relatively recent development, but it is also evidence of the fact that the long-standing stigma associated with anomalous experiences still discourages individuals from sharing details of their encounters. A supernatural or paranormal experience is so foreign to secular worldviews that it often cannot be reconciled with them. Adding to the sense that these sleep phenomena are pathological, health professionals only rarely encounter patients with (disclosed) night-mare concerns—and then only when the experiences are sufficiently distressing and anxiety-provoking to prompt individuals to seek medical care. Lack of information about sleep paralysis still causes confusion, misdiagnosis, and needless suffering.

It has only been during the last two decades that the night-mare has begun to reemerge as a significant figure in American culture—one that can also be recognized by biomedicine, when the entity is conceptualized as sleep paralysis with hypnic hallucinations. From the night-mare's increasingly widespread presence on the Internet and in social media to appearances in magazine articles, literary fiction, television,[1] and film,[2] the terrifying phenomenon is gradually becoming more widely acknowledged. Popular media representations of sleep paralysis reflect the growing awareness of the general population, but they also function to introduce cultural and biological frameworks to terrified and confused first-time experiencers. In an atmosphere of secular skepticism, isolated night-mare sufferers are overwhelmed with relief when their experiences are recognized and accepted. "I'm just glad I stumbled across this group, maybe I won't feel so crazy! You know the way friends and family look at you when you recall what happens?" (Internet posting, ASP-L). It seems likely that sentiments such as these will remain pervasive for some time.

We have learned a tremendous amount about the nature of the night-mare in recent years, but much remains to be explained. There are obvious areas for development, such as research into means of preventing and coping with night-mares (that move beyond changes in sleep position and attempts at toe wiggling), but the list of opportunities for future investigation is varied. Candidates for study include the night-mare's role in community formation, memory development, trauma and coping, religion and spirituality, the nocebo, and mind-body interactions.

The night-mare can provide insight into group development, particularly in the context of virtual communities. The event clearly contributes to a unique sense of shared experience among diverse individuals who seem to have little in common, except for their anomalous nocturnal encounters. Now that communities are no longer bound by geographic locality, will cultural understandings of sleep paralysis develop and evolve differently than they have in the past? How will interpretations of the night-mare function in the virtual spaces that facilitate the formation of online communities? In terms of memory, experiencers note that night-mare encounters are more "real" than waking reality and characteristically leave a deep psychic impression that is felt for decades. How is the night-mare encounter etched in memory in such a way that details can be realistically recalled (and relived) many years later? Regarding stress and coping, in some contexts, night-mares are so terrifying that they meet the clinical criteria for trauma. The emotionally and physically intense encounters with anomalous entities have lasting psychological effects; they traumatize, as well as replay traumas. What is the relationship of night-mares to past traumas and trauma recall among people from different cultures? What can the night-mare teach us about treating people who have experienced trauma?

The night-mare's role has been viewed as significant in terms of religion and spirituality for thousands of years. At the beginning of the twenty-first century, knowledge of the science of sleep paralysis coexists with spiritual explanations, often in the same individual. Given that natural and supernatural understandings of the night-mare have endured for millennia, this is not surprising. Neurophysiological findings regarding sleep paralysis simply do not supplant spiritual interpretations. Scientific developments do not preempt supernatural understandings of sleep paralysis; often, scientific information is incorporated into the interpretation by the individual experiencer (hence the explanation that alien abductors use sleep paralysis to restrain their victims). Near-death and out-of-body experiences also do not lose their spiritual significance when their neurological characteristics are explained. For many night-mare sufferers, science and spirituality are simply not mutually exclusive. By considering the stable set of core night-mare phenomena across religious and scientific traditions, different understandings of these experiences can be explored. The overwhelming majority of night-mare sufferers are physically and mentally healthy people who experience natural, albeit terrifying, events and who logically attempt to understand them by using the explanations available. Because the night-mare is a highly interpretable event, it provides opportunities to study "traditions of disbelief" as well as belief; the very fact that the night-mare experience remains misunderstood and unacknowledged by the majority of Americans is itself worthy of investigation.

Night-mare accounts challenge many of our categories of thought and conceptualizations of the world. Unlike other unusual events described in earlier times or different cultural settings, however, the night-mare provides researchers with unique insight into a shared physical and, to some extent, psychological and emotional experience. The night-mare is a direct link to the experiences of people in diverse cultures, at different times. It is this universal connection that proves so useful in revealing cultural and historical assumptions of meaning-biology interactions. Systematic study of the night-mare can thus further our understanding of the nocebo, beyond its role in Hmong SUNDS/Brugada syndrome. In one formulation of the night-mare experience, sleep paralysis creates expectations of a nocturnal attack, which are subsequently visualized, thus manifesting and confirming the sleeper's worst fears and creating the night-mare experience. The night-mare itself represents a nocebo phenomenon.

Like the nocebo, the night-mare cannot be categorized using conventional mechanistic models. This challenge reveals yet another reason the experience has long resisted scientific study; it defies traditional categories and the division of academic disciplines. Because the night-mare does not respect the boundaries we have set—between science and religion or body and mind—our thinking must also defy conventional, reductionist models in order to understand the experience as fully as possible. Ironically, the night-mare, with its destabilizing of accepted scientific wisdom, can help us as we refine a dynamic model of the interplay between biology and culture.

After enduring for more than five thousand years, there is no indication that the night-mare will ever loosen its tenacious grip. This phenomenon that has afflicted human beings and plagued our sleep from earliest antiquity until the present day is not only a part of our heritage, but it is, apparently, a permanent companion. The night-mare—a link between our biological and cultural selves—will persist.

NOTES

INTRODUCTION

1. Autopsies conflict with the traditional Hmong belief that bodies must remain whole, even in death, to facilitate reincarnation. In the United States, however, autopsies are typically required in cases of unexpected and unexplained deaths. Tissue samples, and occasionally the entire heart, were removed from sudden unexpected death victims under the direction of medical examiners. In early cases, some victims' families were not asked for permission to conduct the autopsy and did not receive explanations of the procedures or their consequences: "Some Hmong families upon getting back the corpse of their dead family member [and,] noticing that the body had been cut open, proceeded to open the body and find to their horror that some organs had been removed" (Holtan et al. 1984, 98–99). This poor communication was a factor in the initially strained relationship between many Hmong immigrants and medical practitioners in the United States.

2. A person experiencing a night terror is actually not awake, but in an altered state of consciousness between slow-wave sleep and a waking state.

3. "Flatereres been the develes chapelleyns, that syngen evere *placebo*" (Chaucer 1390, "The Parson's Tale," 617).

CHAPTER 1   CONSISTENCIES: CROSS-CULTURAL PATTERNS

1. *Night-mare* refers both to the experience itself and to the entity that causes the experience—that is, the attacker.

2. During the course of my research, I analyzed first-person accounts such as this one from publicly accessible Internet postings. I have removed author attributions in all citations to protect individuals' privacy.

3. The inability to cry for help is a particularly disturbing feature (described here by the nineteenth-century Scottish physician Robert MacNish, who himself suffered from night-mares):

> In general, during an attack, the person has the consciousness of an utter inability to express his horror by cries. He feels that his voice is half-choked by impending suffocation, and that any exertion of it, farther than a deep sigh or groan, is impossible. Sometimes, however, he concedes that he is battling with prodigious energy, and wonders that the household are not alarmed by his noise. But this is an illusion: those outcries which he fancies himself uttering, are merely obscure moans, forced with difficulty and pain from the stifled penetralia of his bosom. (MacNish 1834, 126)

4. The "sensed presence" is described particularly well by the psychologist and philosopher William James. In *The Varieties of Religious Experience* (in a section entitled "The Reality of the Unseen"), James quotes from a friend's experience:

> It was about September of 1884. . . . Suddenly I felt something come into the room and stay close to my bed. It remained only a minute or two. I did not recognize it by any ordinary sense, and yet there was a horrible "sensation" connected with it. It stirred something more at the roots of my being than any ordinary perception. The feeling had something of the quality of a very large tearing vital pain spreading chiefly over the chest, but within the organism—and yet the feeling was not pain so much as abhorrence. At all events, something was present with me, and I knew its presence far more surely than I had ever known the presence of any fleshly living creature. I was conscious of its departure as of its coming; an almost instantaneously swift going through the door, and the "horrible sensation" disappeared. (James 1902, 59)

5. As psychoanalyst Ernest Jones notes, the different naturalistic hypotheses fall fairly distinctly into two categories. "On the one hand sources of peripheral irritation, which consist almost exclusively of various indigestible foods, are made to play the chief part in the production of the malady; on the other various mechanical sources of embarrassment to the circulation and respiration, principally a distended stomach and a constrained posture, are asserted to be the efficient agents and to act by bringing about a supply to the brain of non-aerated blood" (Jones 1931, 35–36).

6. Some chronic sufferers appear to reorganize their cognitions in a "calming" way (e.g., "this is just my mind playing tricks"), but many people continue to struggle with the problem and cannot totally discount the possibility that these are "physical events in reality, which are simply beyond the reach of current scientific knowledge" (Uhde, Cortese, and Vedeniapin 2009).

7. The empirical standard for postings is emphasized on the Your Ghost Stories Web site: "If you think dark psychics, men in black, witches, bigfoot, the illuminati or the lizard people are making your life miserable, please seek psychiatric help. Before opening yourself to the paranormal world, I believe it's important to first master critical thinking and reason, and I have no patience with superstition."

8. This work on alien abduction experiences emerged from research that McNally and Clancy had originally undertaken to study women claiming to have recovered memories of childhood sexual abuse. Although the researchers had already found that women who recovered abuse memories were more likely to exhibit "memory distortion," they acknowledge that real traumatic abuse experiences might themselves trigger distorted memories. For purposes of scientific comparison, Clancy and McNally decided to study memory distortion in people who report recovered memories of traumatic events that the researchers did not believe had actually occurred: abduction by space aliens.

9. This argument is reminiscent of one that philosopher Stephen T. Katz made in explaining how mystical experiences are commensurate with cultural understandings. Katz writes that the mystic's life is permeated with the concepts, values, and images of his culture, "which there is no reason to believe he leaves behind in his experience. Rather, these images, beliefs, symbols, and rituals define in advance, what the experience he wants to have, and which he then does have, will be like" (Katz 1978, 33).

10. Folklorists examine groups that organize themselves around shared *dis*beliefs, as well as groups that organize themselves around shared beliefs. As the philosopher and

writer Colin Wilson put it, in his characterization of the views of Charles Fort: "People with a psychological need to *believe* in marvels are no more prejudiced and gullible than people with a psychological need *not* to believe in marvels" (Wilson 2006, 199).

11. The issue of hypnotherapy's role in accounts of alien abductions has been dealt with extensively in the UFO literature by writers representing all viewpoints (e.g., Jacobs 1992; Klass 1988), as well as more broadly in the literature on recovered or false memories (Spanos 1996).

CHAPTER 2   CONTINUITIES: A TRANSHISTORICAL BESTIARY

1. *The Alphabet of Ben Sira* is written in the style of a Biblical commentary and tells the story of the conception, birth, and early education of the "prophet" Ben Sira. The text is intriguing because of its irreverent tone, especially in its treatment of various Biblical characters and rabbinic motifs and in its parodies of specific Talmudic passages. Of the many opinions offered on the origin of the text, theologian Norman Bronznick's seems to be the best substantiated. In his introduction to Stern and Mirsky's collection of narratives from classical Hebrew literature, he suggests that "'The Alphabet' may be one of the earliest literary parodies in Hebrew literature, a kind of academic burlesque—perhaps even entertainment for rabbinic scholars themselves— that included vulgarities, absurdities, and the irreverent treatment of acknowledged sancta" (Stern and Mirsky 1998, 168). The section pertaining to Lilith should be considered in light of the fact that *The Alphabet* was known to have been "read as popular entertainment in most rabbinic communities throughout the Middle Ages" (168). For a comprehensive analysis of historical representations of Lilith, see Scerba 1999.

2. Although we do not have equivalent enduring records from the ancient world, it seems likely that there were male night-mare counterparts in the early folk beliefs of women that were not preserved through written records. Over time, ancient folk traditions have been filtered by a dependence on male literacy for their survival. Perhaps the women of the ancient world were equally plagued by male night-mares. Similarly, the presumption that night-mare spirits only attack those of the opposite sex may also be unfounded. An empirical study of the role of gender and sexuality in the nightmare encounter could test the validity of this supposition.

3. Soranos's writings were adapted from Greek into Latin by Caelius Aurelianus—the original text is now lost.

4. Wilhelm Roscher argues that medieval and renaissance depictions of the devil Mephistopheles are connected with the night-mare/Pan demon (1900).

5. See Stewart 2002 for an excellent presentation of the evolution of the erotic dream/night-mare complex; I discuss only a brief portion of his argument.

6. It is important to remember that variations in night-mare accounts may be the result of differences in reporting and not difference in the actual experiences. In some contexts, this may be particularly true of sexual aspects of the encounters.

7. Kramer and Sprenger's approach did not go unchallenged. In the mid-sixteenth century, for example, Johann Weyer wrote against the persecution of witches. His most influential work is *De Praestigiis Daemonum et Incantationibus ac Venificiis* (*On the Illusions of the Demons and on Spells and Poisons*) (1563).

8. A "sugar loaf"—a tall cone with a rounded top—was the traditional form in which refined sugar was stored until granulated and cube sugars were introduced in the late nineteenth century.

9. I have rendered the trial transcripts in contemporary English by standardizing spelling and pronoun use.

10. The fact that one's "scientific" understanding of the night-mare does nothing to reduce the panic of the experience is evident in many researchers' personal accounts. Max Levin, a twentieth-century neurologist, presents one of own experiences in a case report:

> In the attack I know I am in bed but am otherwise not aware of my surroundings. My eyes are closed. I am conscious of complete inability to move, except to breathe. Breathing seems to be labored, so that I have the idea (during the attack) that the blanket is over my mouth, but can do nothing about it. There is extreme discomfort and anxiety. Though I have been interested in sleep paralysis for years and was the first to employ this phrase in the title of an article, never yet has the thought flashed through my mind, "This is only an attack of sleep paralysis; I must have patience, it will soon pass." I seem to hope that relief will come with the next breath, but each breath leaves me still paralyzed. Finally, after half a dozen unsuccessful attempts, on the next breath I feel as if I am making a Herculean effort, and immediately the spell is broken and I am wide awake and in full possession of my faculties. (Levin 1957, 140)

11. In light of the prevailing views regarding the night-mare and consumption of "indigestible foods," it is interesting to note that Fuseli was said to have "supped on raw pork chops that he might dream his picture of the nightmare" (Cunningham 1829, 93).

12. The potential stimulus for Fuseli's *The Nightmare* still interests art historians, who have focused on an aspect of the artist's troubled personal life as motivation. On the back of the 1781 painting is a portrait of Anna Landolt, a woman Fuseli met in Zurich around 1779 and whom he seriously wanted to marry. Her father refused him, though, and she married another man. In a letter, Fuseli speaks of his erotic dreams and sexual fantasies about her (Powell 1973; Frayling 1996).

13. Shelley's mother, Mary Wollstonecraft, had a relationship (not a serious one, though, to Wollstonecraft's disappointment) with Fuseli (Godwin 1798; Todd 2000; Ward 2000).

14. The events of that remarkable Swiss vacation are loosely depicted in Ken Russell's lurid 1986 horror film, *Gothic*, which also includes a scene in which Fuseli's *The Nightmare* comes grotesquely to life.

15. A few brave authors recounted their personal experiences. One night-mare victim was Sir Arthur Conan Doyle, the creator of Sherlock Holmes and an enthusiastic researcher of paranormal phenomena. As he describes in *The Edge of the Unknown*:

> It was in my bedroom in Crowborough. I awakened in the night with the clear consciousness that there was someone in the room and that the presence was not of this world. I was lying with my back to the room, acutely awake, but utterly unable to move. It was physically impossible for me to turn my body and face this visitor. I heard measured footsteps across the room. I was conscious (without seeing it) that someone was bending over me, and then I heard a voice saying in a loud whisper, "Doyle, I come to tell you that I am sorry." A minute later my disability disappeared, and I was able to turn, but all was black darkness and perfectly still. My wife had not awakened, and knew nothing of what had passed. (Doyle 1930, 71–72)

Even today, there are writers who attribute their literary inspiration to the night-mare:

> My mature birth as a writer can actually be attributed in some measure to these sleep disruptions. . . . It was the changes that these episodes wrought upon my

overall sense of psychic stability that led to my mature efforts at fiction writing. The pervasive mood of absolute, unbearable terror and horror that characterized many of my nights began to seep into my daylight hours and plague me with fears that I might be losing my mind. . . . Sleep paralysis is the most dreadful thing you can imagine. The term "soul-searing" comes to mind but hardly does it justice. I wouldn't wish the experience on anybody. But at least it provides useful grist for the mill; you're more likely to write a decent horror story when your entire life has been overtaken to some degree by the experience of horror itself. (Cardin 2006)

CHAPTER 3   THE NIGHT-MARE ON THE ANALYST'S COUCH

1. Maupassant also makes a connection between sleep paralysis and alien abduction, a decidedly contemporary speculation.

2. In "Maupassant's *Le Horla* and the Cultural-Historical Transformation of the Alien," Cheyne provides the most detailed and insightful analysis of the story's sleep paralysis elements that I have read.

3. Jones appeared to have in mind the role of the night-mare in the development of religion—and the Freudian tenet that religion's roots are pathological. Several authors in the nineteenth and early twentieth centuries hypothesized that the night-mare encounter was the source of belief in evil spirits. In 1889, the historian Ludwig Laistner asserted that the *Uralptraum* (primordial night-mare) was the father of all mythology (1889). Anthropologist Edward Clodd wrote of "the intensified form of dreaming called 'nightmare,' when hideous specters sit upon the breast, stopping breath and paralyzing motion, and to which is largely due to the creation of the vast army of nocturnal demons that fill the folklore of the world, and that, under infinite variety of repellent form, have had place in the hierarchy of religions" (1891, 171). Wolfgang Golther, a folklorist, wrote: "The belief in the soul rests in great part on the conception of torturing and oppressing spirits. Only as a gradual extension of this did the belief arise in spirits that displayed other activities than torturing and oppressing. In the first place, however, the belief in spirits took its origin in the Nightmare" (1895, 75–76).

4. "The explanations of this condition still current in medical circles, and which ascribe it to digestive or circulatory disturbances, are probably farther from the truth than any other medical views, and show as little knowledge of the pathogenesis of the condition as was shown in regard to the infection of wounds before Lister's day, or to tuberculosis before Koch's. This is all the stranger since medical practitioners of earlier centuries were well-informed about the sexual origin of the condition. It is one more illustration of how the advance of medicine in the material field during the past century or two has led to the forgetting of much valuable knowledge in the psychopathological field; the sexual origin of Nightmares had to be rediscovered anew in the twentieth century just as did that of Hysteria" (Jones 1931, 75).

5. Jones's comment is reminiscent of the views expressed by Thomas Hobbes in *Leviathan*: "From this ignorance of how to distinguish dreams, and other strong fancies, from vision and sense, did arise the greatest part of the religion of the Gentiles in time past, that worshipped satyrs, fawns, nymphs and the like; and now-a-days the opinion that rude people have of fairies, ghosts, and goblins, and of the power of witches" (Hobbes 1651, 6).

6. "Anxiety is a libidinal impulse which has its origin in the unconscious and is inhibited by the preconscious. When, therefore, the sensation of inhibition is linked with anxiety in a dream, it must be a question of an act of volition which was at one time

capable of generating libido—that is, it must be a question of a sexual impulse" (Freud 1903, 373).

7. Jones continues his interpretation of the perceived sexual aspects of the night-mare: "It is clear that the great rarity with which Nightmare attacks persons who are sleeping in any other posture than the supine or prone one is readily explicable on the psychological view here maintained, for these are the postures in which the love embrace is normally consummated" (Jones 1931, 49–50).

8. Linking the night-mare with male homosexuality has been a remarkably persistent— yet baseless—association in the psychological and psychiatric literature.

9. Ness (1978) reports similar findings to Hufford (1976), but notes a much higher prevalence rate (62 percent compared to Hufford's 17 percent). This discrepancy is most likely due to methodological differences in data collection (see Hufford 1988, 508).

10. Of course, neither the night-mare's common core content nor its frequency of occurrence in the healthy population eliminate the possibility that people with psychiatric illness can also have night-mares or that their experiences may be interpreted differently by them.

11. Sleep paralysis has also been associated with various mental disorders, including bipolar disorder, panic disorder, and other anxiety disorders (Ohayon et al. 1999; Paradis, Friedman, and Hatch 1997; Stores 1998). Studies have suggested, for example, that sleep paralysis is more prevalent among individuals with panic disorder, an anxiety disorder that causes panic attacks (sudden feelings of terror, fast heartbeat, chest pain, breathing difficulty, dizziness) (Bell, Dixie-Bell, and Thompson 1986). There is some data to suggest that this association may vary across ethnic groups; the range of reported rates for sleep paralysis in African Americans with panic disorder is three times the range of rates of sleep paralysis in white European Americans with panic disorder (Paradis and Friedman 2005). Researchers emphasize the importance of factoring in the impact of racism and stress in the assessment and treatment of African Americans with panic disorder, experiences which may, in turn, increase the risk of sleep disturbances (see Friedman and Paradis 2002; Mellman et al. 2008).

12. The researchers appropriately qualify their findings as preliminary, due to issues of sample size and their lack of assessment of symptoms of post-traumatic stress.

13. My own research with Hmong refugees documented a night-mare prevalence rate of 58 percent. This, however, was in a community-based sample; that is, participants were not selected based on their psychiatric characteristics. It is all the more striking, therefore, that the rate of night-mare attacks was so high in a non-clinical population.

CHAPTER 4   THE NIGHT-MARE IN THE SLEEP LAB

1. One of the earliest detailed scientific accounts of sleep paralysis and hypnic hallucinations, including the observation of the sleeper's supine position, appears to be a case history published in 1664 by Isband van Diemerbroeck, a Dutch physician (Van Diemerbroeck 1664; Kompanje 2008). Almost two hundred years later, Edward Binns described an incident of "utter incapacity for motion or speech, difficult respirations, and extreme dread," which he termed a "daymare," because of its occurrence during a nap (1842). Robert MacNish described the event as "nocturnal paralysis" (1834). Silas Weir Mitchell referred to cases of "nocturnal hemiplegia," "night palsy," "nocturnal paralysis," and "sleep numbness" (1876) It was not until 1928 that Kinnier Wilson first used the term that has become the most accepted: sleep paralysis (Wilson 1928).

2. More recent technological innovations, such as portable sleep monitors, have taken the study of sleep and dreaming out of the laboratory and into natural settings. This will undoubtedly continue the progress that has been made thus far in studying sleep in its range of natural settings (Dement and Koenigsberg 2008).

3. The observation that people's eyes move during dream sleep had, of course, been made by people throughout the world countless times before. Aristotle had noted more than two thousand years earlier that "when sleep takes place, such motions (as occur in the waking state) continue, or are even more apparent" (Aristotle 1996, 93).

4. Many folk traditions are based on the assumption that, in addition to human beings, animals are susceptible to night-mare attacks. It is widely believed that night-mare spirits may attack domestic animals, and that they frequently "disturb horses in their stalls, tire them out by night-riding, and plait or tangle their manes" (Kittredge 1956, 219). These traditions may have arisen from observing the REM cycle, with its characteristic twitches and running motions, in sleeping animals.

5. People with a rare condition called REM sleep behavior disorder lack this normal REM paralysis and can act out their dreams, sometimes leading to severe injuries to their sleeping partners (Kryger, Roth, and Dement 2000).

6. An academic example is, perhaps, warranted: "Relaxation of posture muscles can sometimes be observed in students. If a student goes to sleep during a lecture, the posture muscles retain their tension at first, so the student remains upright. In a few minutes the student may move into something resembling REM sleep. The muscles relax, and the student gradually keels over, striking the desk or a nearby classmate. The student usually wakes up confused, having been awakened in the middle of a dream" (Dewey 2007).

7. "The onset of sleep in nearly all primates is often accompanied by the hypnic or hypnagogic jerk, which is a sudden muscle reflexive movement that frequently awakens the sleeper. Although the ultimate cause of the hypnic jerk is unknown, a common hypothesis is that it is an archaic reflex to the brain's misinterpreting the muscle relaxation accompanying the onset of sleep as a signal that the sleeping primate is falling out of a tree. The reflex may also have had selective value by having the sleeper readjust or review his or her sleeping position in the nest or on a branch in order to assure that a fall did not occur" (Coolidge 2006, 11). Coolidge further suggests that "when ancient hominids stopped sleeping in trees and began sleeping on the ground, slow-wave sleep and REM sleep may have expanded, which may have aided the evolution of humans" (Coolidge 2006, 17).

8. This same set of seemingly "naturalistic" precursors is viewed quite differently by people who think of sleep paralysis as based in the paranormal. Extremely frightening "mind invasion" sleep paralysis attacks "are an attempt at possession by malevolent discarnate entities. . . . Spirit possession is a very real phenomenon, which mainly affects those who, because they're stressed, nervous, or depressed, and are therefore leaking vital energy, have rendered themselves psychically vulnerable" (Proud 2009, 265).

9. Jet-lag also seems to be a precipitating factor of sleep paralysis (Snyder 1983).

10. Based on his assertion that prior to the twentieth century, sleep-disruptive work patterns and long hours were the norm for the majority of people in much of Europe, Davies postulates that there may have been a greater incidence of the night-mare in previous centuries. Additionally, "the intense anxiety created by fear of bewitchment in past societies may have further increased the incidence of the nightmare" (Davies 2003, 189).

11. See also Wing et al. 1999 for results from a study conducted in China.

12. I thank Allan Cheyne for this observation.

13. Body motility is typically relatively high prior to entry into REM (Hobson, Spagna, and Malenka 1978). This may be the reason that people who do not normally attempt to sleep supine find themselves in that position so frequently during sleep paralysis.

14. This appears to be yet another example of sleep paralysis forming a rational and empirical basis for some spiritual/supernatural beliefs. Hufford discusses near-death experiences and their connections to sleep paralysis, including the way in which each has been dismissed and suppressed by the psychopathology model. Near-death experiences and night-mares "illustrate the way in which spiritual conviction in many cultures and through much of history was, in fact, robustly cognitive and rational" (Hufford 2009).

15. In referring to near-death experiences, Nelson explains, "People say that because there's a common thread running through them all there must be a spiritual element. . . . I look at that common thread and I see a biological process" (Fox 2006).

CHAPTER 5   THE NIGHT-MARE, TRADITIONAL HMONG CULTURE, AND SUDDEN DEATH

1. It is difficult to confirm demographic details for many of the early SUNDS cases, since most data were categorized based on nationality rather than ethnicity and thus grouped all Laotians (ethnic Lao, Hmong, Khmu, and others) together.

2. Hmong social structure is characterized by unilineal descent along the male line. In this patrilineal system, clan affiliation is traced from the father, and it is forbidden to marry within one's own clan. This is one reason that allegations of "inbreeding" by uninformed SUNDS researchers were so offensive to the American Hmong community.

3. A premise central to folklore study's intellectual history and development is "that ordinary people tend to be underestimated and that their knowledge tends to be discredited by authorities" (Hufford 1994).

4. My preliminary fieldwork had indicated that, although unemployment and welfare utilization were perhaps overrepresented in Stockton's Hmong community when compared with smaller Hmong communities in California and other states (indicating the possibility of more difficult adjustment problems for individuals), other factors made it a particularly good site at which to conduct field research. It had a network of refugee services, including employment and social services; there was a cohesiveness and closeness to the community that made locating potential participants more feasible; and SUNDS deaths had occurred in the city. In 1988, the city of Stockton had a total population of 150,000, including 5,600 Hmong (Yang and North 1988). I conducted fieldwork from January 1990 to March 1991.

5. Writers have speculated (rather unconvincingly) on such origins as Mesopotamia (Savina 1924), Mongolia, and Siberia (Larteguy 1979; Quincy 1995). Most recent work has only touched on the subject superficially and without academic rigor, while earlier efforts were hampered by the agendas of the missionaries and military observers who undertook them.

6. These Hmong beliefs are reminiscent of contemporary Jewish traditions in areas such as Morocco, Kurdistan, and Yemen that Lilith, as a succubus, poses a danger to pregnant women and newborn children, as well as of medieval European Christian traditions regarding the rape of women by incubi.

7. Children's souls are particularly likely to wander off, since they are easily distracted.

8. I am indebted to David Hufford for the insightful methodology that influenced my approach.

9. About one-third of the interviews were conducted in Hmong with the assistance of bilingual Hmong community interpreters.

10. On rare occasions, the night-mare maintains its otherworldly nature but remains, based on the context in which it is experienced and interpreted, nonthreatening. In one example, a Hmong woman described her night-mare encounter as a visit from her recently deceased husband. His visit served to put her mind at ease regarding his well-being. This night-mare experience was one of only three encounters described by the people I interviewed as having a soothing effect and actually reducing the stress of the individual.

11. Learning English did in fact create a unique issue for the first Hmong immigrants. From a context in which a written Hmong language did not exist before one was constructed by Christian missionaries in the 1950s, and in which the vast majority of adults had no need to learn to read or write, the Hmong moved to a society in which literacy and education are prime requisites for success (Johnson 1985).

12. The notable exception was Hmong women's traditional embroidery, known as *paj ntaub* (pronounced "pa ndau") or "flower cloth," which became popular in the United States and afforded Hmong women a source of income that would have been otherwise unobtainable (Peterson 1988).

13. For one of the Hmong letters written in response, see Vang 1987.

14. Ong addresses, for example, the indiscriminate linking of Cambodian immigrants to PTSD and depression (Ong 2003).

15. In studying Xiong's account, Tobin and Friedman suggest that Xiong may be a survivor of SUNDS. Their argument is weakened, however, by the lack of recognition of the features of the night-mare. When Tobin and Friedman assert that Xiong's "sleeping and breathing difficulties" can be seen "as symptoms of the anxiety, depression, and paranoia that threaten all victims of trauma and extreme stress" (1983, 442), they note important background factors but misread what are in fact the classic symptoms of a night-mare attack. Tobin and Friedman argue that, to "nonbelievers" like themselves, the shaman's explanation can only be true in a metaphorical sense: "Automatically we substitute for her word 'spirit' something we believe in: 'unconscious processes'" (1983, 442).

16. Despite the uniformity of opinion among participants regarding the absence of SUNDS deaths in premigration Laos, it is important to note that the forensic diligence to account for unusual death in Laos is not comparable to that of the United States, particularly in the isolated rural villages in which the Hmong lived. Although it is therefore impossible to know with certainty whether SUNDS deaths occurred in Laos, the conviction on the part of Hmong immigrants that the deaths were absent is a significant element in their dichotomization of experience between premigration Laos and post-resettlement America.

17. Lee's description of the "man in black clothes" recalls the "dark figure" of many contemporary experiences detailed in Internet postings.

CHAPTER 6   THE NIGHT-MARE AND THE NOCEBO:
BELIEFS THAT HARM

1. Fifty years later, in the same Harvard Medical School room in which Cannon performed fight-or-flight experiments, cardiologist Herbert Benson found that there was

a counterbalancing mechanism to the stress response, and he termed this opposite state the "relaxation response."

2. Cannon also believed that the physical insults to the individual's body were compounded by social withdrawal from the victim, because those who are "hexed" normally have committed social transgressions. "All people who stand in kinship relation with him withdraw their sustaining support. . . . The organization of his social life is collapsed and, no longer a member of a group, he is alone and isolated. The doomed man is in a situation from which the only escape is by death" (Cannon 1942, 173–174).

3. According to psychoneuroimmunologist Esther M. Sternberg, "At first glance, it is surprising that scientific discoveries over the last 60 years have largely filled out the details of—but not overturned—most of Cannon's proposed explanation of the physiological underpinnings of this phenomenon. On the other hand, it is not surprising when one considers the fact that Cannon's research formed the basis for much of our modern understanding of the physiological response systems involved in linking emotions, such as fear, with illness. . . . Strikingly absent, however, from Cannon's explanation is the hormonal stress response—the cascade of hormones released from the brain, pituitary gland, and adrenal gland within minutes of exposure to any sort of stressor. This is because in 1942, when the article was written, many of these hormones were yet to be discovered." (Sternberg 2002, 1564–1565).

4. Engel is perhaps best known for formulating the biopsychosocial model, which posits that human health and illness are best understood in terms of a combination of biological, psychological, and social factors, rather than exclusively biological ones. During our correspondence in the 1990s, Engel endorsed my approach to "teasing out the human dimensions of Hmong SUNDS, thereby providing a clear picture of the overall organismic challenge these individuals were facing at the time the 'nightmare' reaction occurred and culminated in sudden death. . . . The biomedical perspective is incapable of encompassing such a possibility, indeed, I would put it, disallows even thinking about it" (Engel 1994, personal correspondence).

5. The idea that sudden death can be caused by intense emotional stress is commonplace in folklore. Stith Thompson's *Motif-Index of Folk-Literature* (1955) cites examples of motifs of death caused by broken heart (F1041.1.1), chagrin (F1041.1.3.10), grief (T211.9.1), grief over death (F1041.1.2), meeting a ghost (E265.3), and joy (F1041.1.5). The possibility of sudden death during psychological stress is also widely recognized in medical writings of the eighteenth and nineteenth centuries. Indeed, as Engel notes, it was only in the late nineteenth century that such notions fell into disrepute. "Physicians embraced the more rational and objective view that 'cause of death' was to be established at the necropsy table and in the laboratory. Since then consideration of the relationship between emotion and sudden death has virtually disappeared from the medical literature, or at best the idea is greeted with skepticism if not incredulity or downright ridicule" (Engel 1971, 772).

6. Not all of the early research into psychogenic death focused on specific disorders. Researchers studied, for example, the increased mortality that exists among widows and widowers (e.g., Jacobs and Ostfeld 1977; Parkes, Benjamin, and Fitzgerald 1969). Mortality rates for widowed people in every age group were found to be higher than for married people. Research suggested that widowed individuals have a greater risk of dying than married people of a similar age and that this excess risk is greater for men. Bereavement studies were among the first to assert, in biomedical terms, that emotional stress could play a major role in elevated risk of death.

7. Although the reason for this gender discrepancy remains a biomedical mystery, scientists believe that "there is probably a complex interplay of age- and gender-dependent genetic and other precipitating and/or modulating factors (e.g., circadian variations of sympatho-vagal balance, hormones, metabolic factors) that cause tachyarrhythmias or diminish an individual "ventricular fibrillation reserve" at a particular point of time in life" (Lars 2007, 422).

8. SCN5A mutations have now been found in other sudden-death syndromes, including some cases of sudden infant death syndrome, or SIDS (Ackerman, Siu, and Sturner 2002).

9. When Marley's ghost queries, "Why do you doubt your senses?" Scrooge replies, "Because . . . a little thing affects them. A slight disorder of the stomach makes them cheats. You may be an undigested bit of beef, a blot of mustard, a crumb of cheese, a fragment of an underdone potato. There's more of gravy than of grave about you, whatever you are!" (Dickens 2010, 15).

10. Sudden nocturnal death is polysemic, as well. A sudden or swift death (*pokkuri shinu*) is described as an ideal way to die by many elderly Japanese (Traphgan 2000). In Japan, thousands of elderly people visit the Buddhist temple at Kichidenji, the best known of the *pokkuri-dera*, or "temples of sudden death." They pray for a sudden, unexpected death (without suffering from a prolonged illness), and they pray that they remain healthy until the moment of death. "The Japanese are the longest-lived nation in the world, and the prospect of extended illness in old age is not an appealing one. Even a sudden death in the night can be seen as a blessing rather than a curse" (Hambling 2006). "Although many of the Japanese elderly prefer to be cared for by their family and expect their family to care for them, they also feel that they do not want to be a burden. A *pokkuri* death is thought to protect the elderly from being a care giving burden" (Takahashi 2009).

11. There seems to be a range of variation in individual "meaning responses" to external influences that may make some people more likely to experience strong nocebo or placebo effects (Spiegel 1997). In addition, "the meaning response appears to be stronger for some ailments, such as nausea or pain, than others, such as toxin-induced diarrhea or inflammation related to an insect bite. Interestingly, . . . many indigenous belief systems categorize illnesses into those that are more or less spiritual in aspect, perhaps reflecting awareness of the meaning response" (Whitaker 2006, 340).

12. Annual statistics regarding Laotian arrivals were obtained from Linda Gordon, chief statistician at the Office for Refugee Resettlement.

13. Although the Hmong in the United States were in the process of adapting to new conditions, many may not yet have had adequate resources in their new cultural contexts to ease tremendous stress and anxiety. As Jacques Lemoine reports, "The strangest thing is that many of the [SUNDS] cases we investigated were people who had already adapted or were adapting themselves. They had given up their traditional protection" (Lemoine 1986, 347). In terms of traditional beliefs and behaviors, many Hmong were apparently caught between no longer being able to practice their traditional religion and not yet being fully comfortable with recently adapted or newly acquired ones. For many Hmong, traditional modes of dealing with *dab tsog* were unavailable or, as was the case with many of the Christian Hmong I interviewed, hesitatingly rejected.

14. The psychological stress is thus multifactorial and more contingent than simply the terror of *dab tsog*, although that fear can be enormous. Some otherwise accurate

characterizations of my research have oversimplified this point (e.g., Benson and Stark 1996; Benson 1997; Greer 2002).

CONCLUSION

1. The Lifetime Network movie *Nightmare* is a television melodrama about a sleep researcher: "A graduate student begins to experience sleep paralysis and has visions of an evil presence that seem all too real" (Lifetime 2007). *The Nightmare* (Gray and Gray 2008) and *Your Worst Nightmare: Supernatural Assault* (Taitt and Barnes 2008) are representative of recent television documentaries.

2. Although misattributed to "dreams" in the following account, Wes Craven's inspiration for his 1984 horror film, *A Nightmare on Elm Street*, is clearly *dab tsog*:

> Long fascinated by dreams and the role they play in the unconscious, Craven had come across a remarkable story about immigrants from Laos who had died, apparently as a result of horrific nightmares. Evidently hundreds of Laotians— particularly those known as the Hmong—had died from a disorder that is now known as SUNDS, the Sudden Unexpected Nocturnal Death Syndrome. The first such death was reported 1977, and at the time of Craven's interest in these cases, researchers could not determine "what it is that is killing these seemingly healthy people in their sleep" (Adler 1991). This idea—grim and tragic as it was—fasci- nated Wes Craven, appealing to his ongoing interest in dreams and dreamers and his love of producing cinematic horror. Craven's new movie took as a point of departure the idea of dreams that kill and created a character who would, himself, become a symbol of horror and popular culture: Freddy Krueger. (Blitz and Krasniewicz 2007, 16)

Other night-mare-themed movies include *Incubus* (1965), an American film about a pair of succubi who are seeking additional victims (performed entirely in Esperanto, directed by Leslie Stevens, creator of *The Outer Limits*, and starring a pre–*Star Trek* William Shatner); *Gothic* (1986), an American film depicting a fictionalized account of Mary Shelley's visit with Lord Byron by Lake Geneva and the famous challenge to create a horror story, which ultimately led to Mary Shelley's writing *Frankenstein* and John Polidori's writing *The Vampyre*; and *Sleep Paralysis* (2004), an Australian film about a children's book author whose increasingly intense nocturnal attacks threaten not only to end her successful career, but her life.

REFERENCES

Ackerman, M. J., B. L. Siu, W. Q. Sturner, D. J. Tester, C. R. Valdivia, J. C. Makielski, and J. A. Towbin. 2002. Postmortem molecular analysis of SCN5A defects in sudden infant death syndrome. *Journal of the American Medical Association* 286(18): 2264–2269.

Adler, Shelley R. 1991. Sudden unexpected nocturnal death syndrome among Hmong immigrants: Examining the role of the "nightmare." *The Journal of American Folklore* 104(411): 54–71.

Adler, Shelley R. 1994. Ethnomedical pathogenesis and Hmong immigrants' sudden nocturnal deaths. *Culture, Medicine, and Psychiatry* 18(1): 23–59.

American Psychiatric Association. 1994. *Diagnostic and statistical manual of mental disorders: DSM-IV.* 4th ed. Washington, DC: American Psychiatric Association.

American Psychiatric Association. 2000. *Diagnostic and statistical manual of mental disorders: DSM-IV-TR.* Washington, DC: American Psychiatric Association.

American Refugee Committee. 1989. Update: Sudden unexplained death syndrome among Southeast Asian refugees. *Refugee Health Issues Quarterly* 4(2): 1, 3.

Appelle, S. 2000. Ufology and academia: The UFO phenomenon as a scholarly discipline. In *UFOs and abductions: Challenging the borders of knowledge,* ed. D. M. Jacobs, 7–30. Lawrence, KS: University Press of Kansas.

Arikawa, H., D. I. Templer, R. Brown, W. G. Cannon, and S. Thomas-Dodson. 1999. The structure and correlates of kanashibari. *Journal of Psychology* 133(4): 369–375.

Aristotle. 1996. *On sleep and dreams.* London: Aris & Phillips.

Armstrong, K. 1994. *A history of god: The 4000-year quest of Judaism, Christianity, and Islam.* New York: Ballantine.

Artemidorus. 1975. *Interpretation of dreams: Oneirocritica.* Trans. R. J. White. Park Ridge, NJ: Noyes Press.

Aserinsky, E. 1996. The discovery of REM sleep. *Journal of the History of the Neurosciences* 5(3): 213–227.

Augustine. 1972. *De civitate dei (City of God).* Trans. H. Bettenson. Harmondsworth, England: Penguin Books. (Orig. pub. c. fifth century CE)

Awadalla, A., G. Al-Fayez, M. Harville, H. Arikawa, M. E. Tomeo, D. I. Templer, and R. Underwood. 2004. Comparative prevalence of isolated sleep paralysis in Kuwaiti, Sudanese, and American college students. *Psychological Reports* 95(1): 317–322.

Barber, Paul. 1988. *Vampires, burial, and death: Folklore and reality.* New Haven, CT and London: Yale University Press.

Baron, R. C., and R. H. Kirschner. 1983. Sudden night-time death among South-East Asians too. *The Lancet* 1(8327): 764.

Bass, Ellen, and Laura Davis. 1988 *The courage to heal: A guide for women survivors of child sexual abuse.* New York: HarperCollins.

Beinfield, Harriet, and Efrem Korngold. 1991. *Between heaven and earth: A guide to Chinese medicine.* New York and Toronto: Ballantine Books.

Belanti, J., M. Perera, and K. Jagadheesan. 2008. Phenomenology of near-death experiences: A cross-cultural perspective. *Transcultural Psychiatry* 45(1): 121–133.

Bell, Carl C., Bambade Shakoor, Belinda Thompson, Donald Dew, Eugene Hughley, Raymond Mays, and Kumea Shorter-Gooden. 1984. Prevalence of isolated sleep paralysis in black subjects. *Journal of the National Medical Association* 76(5): 501–508.

Bell, Carl C., Dora D. Dixie-Bell, and Belinda Thompson. 1986. Further studies on the prevalence of isolated sleep paralysis in black subjects. *Journal of the National Medical Association* 78(7): 649–659.

Benson, Herbert. 1997. The nocebo effect: History and physiology. *Preventive Medicine* 26(5 Pt 1): 612–615.

Benson, Herbert, and Marg Stark. 1996. *Timeless healing: The power and biology of belief.* New York: Scribner.

Binns, E. 1842. *The anatomy of sleep; or, the art of procuring sound and refreshing slumber at will.* London: J. Churchill.

Bissinger, H. G. 1981. "More cities report death syndrome." *St. Paul Pioneer Press,* F1: 4. 6 February.

Blackmore, Susan. 1994. Alien abduction: The inside story. *New Scientist* (19 November): 29–31.

Blackmore, Susan. 1998. Abduction by aliens or sleep paralysis? *Skeptical Inquirer* 22(3): 23–28.

Bliatout, Bruce Thowpaou. 1982. *Hmong sudden unexpected nocturnal death syndrome: A cultural study.* Portland, OR: Sparkle Publications.

Bliatout, Bruce Thowpaou. 2003. Social and spiritual explanations of depression and nightmares. In *Healing by heart: Clinical and ethical case stories of Hmong families and Western providers,* eds. Kathleen A. Culhane-Pera, Dorothy E. Vawter, Phua Xiong, Barbara Babbitt, and Mary M. Solberg, 209–215. Nashville, TN: Vanderbilt University Press.

Blitz, Michael, and Louise Krasniewicz. 2007. *Johnny Depp: A biography.* Westport, CT: Greenwood Press.

Bloom, J. D., and R. D. Gelardin. 1976. Uqamairineq and uqumanigianiq: Eskimo sleep paralysis. *Arctic* 29 (1): 20–26.

Boiadjiev, Tzotcho, and Barbara Müller. 2003. *Die Nacht im Mittelalter.* Würzburg: Königshausen and Neumann.

Bond, John. 1751. *Dissertatio medica inauguralis de incubo.* Edinburgh: T. and W. Ruddimannos.

Bond, John. 1753. *An essay on the incubus, or night-mare.* London: D. Wilson and T. Durham.

Boyer, Paul, and Stephen Nissenbaum, eds. 1977. *The Salem witchcraft papers: Verbatim transcripts of the legal documents of the Salem witchcraft outbreak of 1692.* 3 vols. New York: Da Capo Press. (Orig. pub. 1938.)

Bremmer, Rolf H., Thomas S. B. Johnston, and Oebele Vries, eds. 1998. *Approaches to old Frisian philology.* Amsterdam and Atlanta, GA: Rodopi.

Brodsky, M. A., D. A. Sato, L. T. Iseri, L. J. Wolff, and B. J. Allen. 1987. Ventricular tachyarrhythmia associated with psychological stress: The role of the sympathetic nervous system. *Journal of the American Medical Association* 257(15): 2064–2067.

Brody, J. 1990. "Mysterious Disease Stalks Asian Refugees." *The Orange County Register,* 9 April, 12.

Brugada, P., and J. Brugada. 1992. Right bundle branch block, persistent ST segment elevation, and sudden cardiac death: A distinct clinical and electrocardiographic syndrome. A multicenter report. *Journal of the American College of Cardiology* 20(6): 1391–1396.

Bullard, Thomas E. 1989. UFO abduction reports: The supernatural kidnap narrative returns in technological guise. *Journal of American Folklore* 102(404): 147–170.

Buzzi, G., and F. Cirignotta. 2000. Isolated sleep paralysis: A Web survey. *Sleep Research Online* 3(2): 61–66.

Cannon, Walter Bradford. 1915. *Bodily changes in pain, hunger, fear, and rage.* New York and London: D. Bradford and Company.

Cannon, Walter Bradford. 1942. "Voodoo" death. *American Anthropologist* 44(new series): 169–181.

Cardin, Matt. 2006 "Fun with nocturnal assault." The Teeming Brain. http://theteemingbrain.wordpress.com/2006/10/25/fun-with-nocturnal-assault

Carlson, Eugene. 1981. "Refugee influx to some areas straining budgets, good will." *Wall Street Journal,* 3 November, 37.

Centers for Disease Control. 1988. Update: Sudden unexplained death syndrome among Southeast Asian refugees—United States. *Morbidity and Mortality Weekly Report* 37(37): 568–570.

Cerquone, Joseph. 1986. *Refugees from Laos: In harm's way.* Washington, DC: U.S. Committee for Refugees.

Cha, Dia. 2003. *Hmong American concepts of health, healing, and conventional medicine.* New York: Routledge.

Chambers, Paul. 1999. *Sex and the paranormal.* London: Blandford.

Chaucer, Geoffrey. 1957. *The Canterbury tales.* Boston, MA: Houghton Mifflin. (Orig. pub. c. 1390.)

Cheyne, James Allan. n.d. Maupassant's *le horla* and the cultural-historical transformation of the alien. http://watarts.uwaterloo.ca/~acheyne/LeHorla.pdf

Cheyne, James Allan. 2001. The ominous numinous: Sensed presence and "other" hallucinations. *Journal of Consciousness Studies* 8(5–7): 133–150.

Cheyne, James Allan. 2002. Situational factors affecting sleep paralysis and associated hallucinations: Position and timing effects. *Journal of Sleep Research* 11(2): 169–177.

Cheyne, James Allan. 2005. Sleep paralysis episode frequency and number, types, and structure of associated hallucinations. *Journal of Sleep Research* 14(3): 319–324.

Cheyne, James Allan, and Todd A. Girard. 2008. The body unbound: Vestibular-motor hallucinations and out-of-body experiences. *Cortex* 45(2): 201–215.

Cheyne, James Allan, Ian R. Newby-Clark, and Steve D. Rueffer. 1999. Relations among hypnagogic and hypnopompic experiences associated with sleep paralysis. *Journal of Sleep Research* 8(4): 313–317.

Cheyne, James Allan, Steve D. Rueffer, and Ian R. Newby-Clark. 1999. Hypnagogic and hypnopompic hallucinations during sleep paralysis: Neurological and cultural construction of the night-mare. *Consciousness and Cognition* 8(3): 319–337.

Chiu, Jeannie. 2004. I salute the spirit of my communities: Autoethnographic innovations in Hmong American literature. *College Literature* 31(3): 43–69.

Chiu, Monica. 2004–05. Medical, racist, and colonial constructions of power: Creating the Asian American patient and the cultural citizen in Anne Fadiman's *The Spirit Catches You and You Fall Down. Hmong Studies Journal* 5: 1–36.

Clancy, Susan A. 2005. *Abducted: How people come to believe they were kidnapped by aliens.* Cambridge, MA: Harvard University Press.

Clark, S. E., and E. F. Loftus. 1996. The construction of space alien abduction memories. *Psychological Inquiry* 7(2): 140–143.

Clifford, James. 2002. *The predicament of culture: 20th-century ethnography, literature, and art.* Cambridge, MA: Harvard University Press.

Clodd, Edward. 1891. *Myths and dreams*. London: Chatto and Windus.

Coolidge, Frederick L. 2006. *Dream interpretation as a psychotherapeutic technique*. Abingdon, UK: Radcliffe Publishing.

Cunningham, Alan. 1829. *The lives of the most eminent British painters*. Vol. 2. London.

Curry, Bill. 1981. "'Nightmare syndrome'? Deaths of Laos refugees puzzle officials." *Los Angeles Times*, 26 February, 16.

Dacome, Lucia. 2004. "To what purpose does it think?": Dreams, sick bodies, and confused minds in the Age of Reason. *History of Psychiatry* 15(4): 395–416.

Dao, Yang. 1982. Why did the Hmong leave Laos? In *The Hmong in the West: Observations and reports: Papers of the 1981 Hmong research conference, University of Minnesota*, eds. B. T. Downing and D. P. Olney. Minneapolis, MN: Southeast Asian Refugee Studies Project, Center for Urban and Regional Affairs, University of Minnesota.

Darwin, Erasmus. 1791. *The botanic garden; a poem, in two parts*. London: J. Johnson.

Davidson, Keay. 1981. "Puzzle of Laotian refugee deaths is probed in S.D." *Los Angeles Times*, 12 September, SD-A1.

Davies, Owen. 1996. Hag-riding in nineteenth-century west country England and modern Newfoundland: An examination of an experience-centered witchcraft tradition. *Folk Life* 35: 36–53.

Davies, Owen. 2003. The nightmare experience, sleep paralysis, and witchcraft accusations. *Folklore* 114(2): 181–203

de Jong, J. T. 2005. Cultural variation in the clinical presentation of sleep paralysis. *Transcultural Psychiatry* 42(1): 78–92.

Dement, William C., and Robert Koenigsberg. 2008. Winds of change in sleep medicine. *Sleep Review*, http://www.sleepreviewmag.com/issues/articles/2008–06_07.asp

Desan, Christine. 1983. A change of faith for Hmong refugees. *Cultural Survival Quarterly* 7: 45–48.

Devinsky, O., E. Feldmann, K. Burrowes, and E. Bromfield. 1989. Autoscopic phenomena with seizures. *Archives of Neurology* 46(10): 1080–1088.

Dewey, Russell A. 2007. Psychology: An introduction. http://www.intropsych.com

Dickens, Charles. 2010. *A Christmas Carol in Prose, Being a Ghost Story of Christmas*. London: Cecil Palmer. (Orig. pub. 1843)

Dolan, Terence Patrick. 2006. *A dictionary of Hiberno-English: The Irish use of English*. Dublin: Gill and Macmillan.

Donnelly, Francis X. 2005. "Culture shock, poverty plague Hmong in Michigan." *Detroit News*, 12 April.

Donnelly, Nancy D. 1994. *Changing lives of refugee Hmong women*. Seattle, WA: University of Washington Press.

Dorais, Louis-Jacques. 1997. *Quaqtaq: Modernity and identity in an Inuit community*. Toronto and Buffalo, NY: University of Toronto Press.

Douglas, N. J., and O. Polo. 1994. Pathogenesis of obstructive sleep apnoea/hypopnoea syndrome. *The Lancet* 344(8923): 653–655.

Doyle, Arthur Conan. 1930. *The edge of the unknown*. London: J. Murray.

Dror, Otniel E. 2004. "Voodoo death": Fantasy, excitement, and the untenable boundaries of biomedical science. In *The politics of healing: Essays in the twentieth-century history of North American alternative medicine*, ed. R. D. Johnston, 71–81. London and New York: Routledge.

Druffel, Ann. 1998. *How to defend yourself against alien abduction*. New York: Three Rivers Press.

Ducie, Earl of. 1888. Exhibition of three "mare-stanes," or "hag-stones." *Journal of the Anthropological Institute of Great Britain and Ireland* 17: 134–137.

Eaker, E. D., J. Pinsky, and W. P. Castelli. 1992. Myocardial infarction and coronary death among women: Psychosocial predictors from a 20-year follow-up of women in the Framingham study. *American Journal of Epidemiology* 135(8): 854–864.

Eastwell, H. D. 1982. Voodoo death and the mechanism for dispatch of the dying in east Arnhem, Australia. *American Anthropologist* 84(1): 5–18.

Elliott, D. 1999. *Fallen bodies: Pollution, sexuality and demonology.* Philadelphia: University of Pennsylvania Press.

Emmons, C. F. 1982. *Chinese ghosts and ESP: A study of paranormal beliefs and experiences.* Metuchen, NJ: Scarecrow Press.

Engel, George L. 1971. Sudden and rapid death during psychological stress: Folklore or folk wisdom? *Annals of Internal Medicine* 74(5): 771–782.

Ethelberg, S. 1956. Sleep-paralysis or post-dormitial chalastic fits in cortical lesion of the frontal pole. *Acta Psychiatrica Scandinavica. Supplementum* 108: 121–130.

Everett, Henry C. 1963. Sleep Paralysis in Medical Students. *Journal of Nervous and Mental Disease* 136(3): 283–287.

Ewen, C. L'Estrange. 1933. *Witchcraft and demonism.* London: Heath Cranton.

Faderman, Lillian, and Ghia Xiong. 1998. *I begin my life all over: The Hmong and the American immigrant experience.* Boston: Beacon Press.

Fadiman, Anne. 1997. *The spirit catches you and you fall down: A Hmong child, her American doctors, and the collision of two cultures.* New York: Farrar, Straus, and Giroux.

Firestone, Melvin. 1985. The "old hag": Sleep paralysis in Newfoundland. *Journal of Psychoanalytic Anthropology* 8: 47–66.

Fitzgerald, F. Scott. 1922. *The beautiful and damned.* London: Collins.

Fletcher, C., and Kirmayer, L. J. 1997. Spirit work: Nunavimmiut experiences of affliction and healing. *Etudes/Inuit/Studies* 21(1–2): 189–208.

Folkard, Simon, Ruth Condon, and M. Herbert. 1984. Night shift paralysis. *Experientia* 40(5): 510–512.

Folkard, Simon, and Ruth Condon. 1987. Night shift paralysis in air traffic control officers. *Ergonomics* 30(9): 1353–1363.

Foster, George M. 1973. Dreams, character, and cognitive orientation in Tzintzuntzan. *Ethos* 1(1): 106–121.

Foulkes, David, and Gerald Vogel. 1965. Mental activity at sleep onset. *Journal of Abnormal Psychology* 70(4): 231–243.

Fox, Douglas. 2006. Light at the end of the tunnel. *New Scientist* (17 October): 48–50.

Frayling, Christopher. 1996. *Nightmare: The birth of horror.* London: BBC Books.

Freud, Sigmund. 1903. *The interpretation of dreams.* Trans. A. A. Brill. New York: MacMillan. (Orig. pub. 1900.)

Friedman, Steven, and Cheryl Paradis. 2002. Panic disorder in African-Americans: Symptomatology and isolated sleep paralysis. *Culture, Medicine, and Psychiatry* 26(2): 179–198.

Fukuda, Kazuhiko. 1993. One explanatory basis for the discrepancy of reported prevalences of sleep paralysis among healthy respondents. *Perceptual and Motor Skills* 77(3): 803–807.

Fukuda, Kazuhiko, Robert D. Ogilvie, Lisa Chilcott, Ann-Marie Vendittelli, and Tomoka Takeuchi. 1998. The prevalence of sleep paralysis among Canadian and Japanese college students. *Dreaming* 8(2): 59–66.

Garcia-Touchard, A., V. K. Somers, T. Kara, J. Nykodym, A. Shamsuzzaman, P. Lanfranchi, and M. J. Ackerman. 2007. Ventricular ectopy during REM sleep: Implications for nocturnal sudden cardiac death. *Nature Clinical Practice Cardiovascular Medicine* 4(5): 284–288.

Godwin, William. 1798. *Memoirs of the author of a vindication of the rights of woman*. London: Joseph Johnson.

Golther, Wolfgang. 1895. *Handbuch der Germanischen Mythologie*. Trans. E. Jones. Leipzig: S. Hirzel.

Goode, G. B. 1962. Sleep paralysis. *Archives of Neurology* 6(3): 228–234.

Gray, Adam, and Andrew Gray. 2008. *The nightmare*. DVD. Directed by the Gray Brothers. New York: Paradocs Productions.

Grayman, J. H., M. J. Good, and B. J. Good. 2009. Conflict nightmares and trauma in Aceh. *Culture, Medicine, and Psychiatry* 33(2): 290–312.

Greer, John Michael. 2002. *Monsters*. St. Paul, MN: Llewellyn Publications.

Hahn, Robert A. 1995. *Sickness and healing: An anthropological perspective*. New Haven, CT: Yale University Press.

Hahn, Robert A. 1997. The nocebo phenomenon: Concept, evidence, and implications for public health. *Preventive Medicine* 26(5): 607–611.

Hahn, Robert, and Arthur Kleinman. 1983. Belief as pathogen, belief as medicine: "Voodoo death" and the "placebo phenomenon" in anthropological perspective. *Medical Anthropology Quarterly* 14(3): 6–19.

Halifax, Joan. 1991. *Shamanic voices: A survey of visionary narratives*. New York: Penguin.

Hambling, David. 2006. "Nightmare death syndrome." Fortean Times: The World of Strange Phenomena, http://www.forteantimes.com/strangedays/medicalbag/335/nightmare_death_syndrome.html

Hamilton-Merritt, Jane. 1999. *Tragic mountains: The Hmong, the Americans, and the secret war for Laos, 1942–1992*. Bloomington, IN: Indiana University Press.

Hardy, Thomas. 1896. *The Wessex tales*. London: Osgood, McIlvaine, and Co.

Harrington, Anne. 2008. *The cure within: A history of mind-body medicine*. New York: W. W. Norton.

Heimbach, Ernest E. 1979. White Hmong-English Dictionary. Ithaca, NY: Cornell Southeast Asia Program.

Hemingway, Ernest. 1936. *The snows of Kilimanjaro: A long story*. Chicago: Esquire Inc.

Her, Vincent K. 2005. Hmong cosmology: Proposed model, preliminary insights. *Hmong Studies Journal* 6: 1–25.

Herodotus. 1954. *The Histories*. Trans. Aubrey de Selincourt. London and New York: Penguin Books.

Herr, Paul Pao. 1990. "Don't call Hmong refugees primitive." *New York Times*, 29 November, A28.

Hinton, Devon E., and Byron Good. 2009. *Culture and panic disorder*. Stanford, CA: Stanford University Press.

Hinton, Devon E., A. L. Hinton, Vuth Pich, J. R. Loeum, and Mark H. Pollack. 2009. Nightmares among Cambodian refugees: The breaching of concentric ontological security. *Culture, Medicine, and Psychiatry* 33(2): 219–265.

Hinton, Devon E., David J. Hufford, and Laurence J. Kirmayer. 2005. Culture and sleep paralysis. *Transcultural Psychiatry* 42(1): 5–10.

Hinton, Devon E., Vuth Pich, Dara Chhean, and Mark H. Pollack. 2005. "The ghost pushes you down": Sleep paralysis-type panic attacks in a Khmer refugee population. *Transcultural Psychiatry* 42(1): 46–77.

Hishikawa, Yasuo. 1976. Sleep paralysis. In *Narcolepsy: Proceedings of the first international symposium on narcolepsy, July 1975, Montpellier, France,* eds. C. Guilleminault, W. C. Dement, and N. Passouant, 97–124. New York: Spectrum Publications.

Hishikawa, Y., and T. Shimizu. 1995. Physiology of REM sleep, cataplexy, and sleep paralysis. *Advances in Neurology* 67: 245–271.

Hobbes, Thomas. 1651. *Leviathan, or, the matter, forme, & power of a common-wealth ecclesiasticall and civill.* London: Andrew Crooke.

Hobson, J. A., T. Spagna, and R. Malenka. 1978. Ethology of sleep studied with time-lapse photography: Postural immobility and sleep-cycle phase in humans. *Science* 201(4362): 1251–1253.

Holder, Desonta. 2007. "Does the fear of dying become a self-fulfilling prophecy for people?" *Oakland Tribune.* 12 November.

Holtan, Neal. 1984. Memorandum to epidemiology discussion group, July 27. In *Immigration history research center, Box 3, Folder 33, University of Minnesota.* Minneapolis, MN.

Holtan, Neal, Dave Carlson, Jean Egbert, Rachel Mielke, and T. Christopher Thao. 1984. *Final report of the SUNDS planning project: A summary of the current state of knowledge about sudden unexpected nocturnal death syndrome occurring in Southeast Asians with recommendations for research and community action.* Saint Paul. MN: Saint Paul-Ramsey Medical Center.

Hooper, Robert. 1811. *Lexicon medicum; a new medical dictionary.* New York: J. and J. Harper.

Hufford, David J. 1976. A new approach to the "old hag": The night-mare tradition reexamined. In *American folk medicine: A symposium,* ed. W. D. Hand. Berkeley, CA: University of California Press.

Hufford, David J. 1982. *The terror that comes in the night: An experience-centered study of supernatural assault traditions.* Philadelphia: University of Pennsylvania Press.

Hufford, David J. 1988. Inclusionism versus reductionism in the study of culture-bound syndromes. *Culture, Medicine, and Psychiatry* 12(4): 503–512.

Hufford, David J. 1994. Folklore and medicine. In *Putting folklore to use,* ed. M. O. Jones, 117–135. Lexington, KY: University Press of Kentucky.

Hufford, David J. 2005. Sleep paralysis as spiritual experience. *Transcultural Psychiatry* 42(1): 11–45.

Hufford, David J. 2009. Visionary spiritual experiences and cognitive aspects of spiritual transformation. *The Global Spiral,* http://www.metanexus.net/magazine/tabid/68/id/10610/Default.aspx

Iber, C., S. Ancoli-Israel, A. I. Chesson, S. F. Quan. 2007. *The AASM Manual for the Scoring of Sleep and Associated Events: Rules, Terminology, and Technical Specifications.* Westchester, IL: American Academy of Sleep Medicine.

Ikeda, T., A. Abe, S. Yusu, K. Nakamura, H. Ishiguro, H. Mera, M. Yotsukura, et al. 2006. The full stomach test as a novel diagnostic technique for identifying patients at risk of Brugada syndrome. *Journal of Cardiovascular Electrophysiology* 17(6): 602–607.

Ingall, Michael. 1984. Southeast Asian refugees of Rhode Island: Psychiatric problems, cultural factors, and nightmare death. *Rhode Island Medical Journal* 67(8): 369–372.

Jacobs, D. 1992. *Secret life: Firsthand, documented accounts of UFO abductions.* New York: Simon and Shuster.

Jacobs, S., and A. Ostfeld. 1977. An epidemiological review of the mortality of bereavement. *Psychosomatic Medicine* 39(5): 344–357.

Jacobsen, Thorkild. 1939. *The Sumerian king list.* Chicago: University of Chicago Press.

Jacobson, C. J., Jr. 2009. The nightmares of Puerto Ricans: An embodied "altered states of consciousness" perspective. *Culture, Medicine, and Psychiatry* 33(2): 266–289.

James I. 2008. *Daemonologie.* Forgotten Books. (Orig. pub. 1597)

James, William. 1902. *The varieties of religious experience: A study in human nature.* New York: Random House.

Jarcho, Saul. 1980. Some lost, obsolete, or discontinued diseases: Serous apoplexy, incubus, and retrocedent ailments. *Transactions and Studies of the College of Physicians of Philadelphia* 2(5): 241–266.

Jiménez-Genchi, Alejandro, Víctor M. Ávila-Rodríguez, Frida Sánchez-Rojas, Blanca E. Vargas Terrez, and Alejandro Nenclares-Portocarrero. 2009. Sleep paralysis in adolescents: The 'a dead body climbed on top of me' phenomenon in Mexico. *Psychiatry and Clinical Neurosciences* 63(4): 546–549.

Johnson, Charles. 1985. *Dab neeg hmoob: Myths, legends, and folktales from the Hmong of Laos.* St. Paul, MN: Macalester College.

Johnson, R. C. 1994. Parallels between recollections of repressed childhood sex abuse, kidnappings by space aliens, and the 1692 Salem witch hunts. *Issues in Child Abuse Accusations* 6(1): 41–47.

Johnson, Steve. 1991. "Strange malady killing Asian men." *San Jose Mercury News,* 18 February, 1A.

Jones, Ernest. 1931. *On the nightmare, the international psycho-analytical library, No. 20.* London: L. & Virginia Woolf at the Hogarth Press, and the Institute of Psycho-analysis.

Jouvet, Michel. 2001. *The paradox of sleep: The story of dreaming.* Trans. L. Garey. Cambridge, MA: MIT Press.

Kaiser, Tamara L. 2004–05. Caught between cultures: Hmong parents in America's sibling society. *Hmong Studies Journal* 5: 1–14.

Katz, Stephen T. 1978. Language, epistemology, and mysticism. In *Mysticism and philosophical analyses,* ed. S. T. Katz, 22–74. London: Sheldon Press.

Kiessling, Nicolas. 1968. Grendel: A new aspect. *Modern Philology* 65(3): 191–201.

Kiessling, Nicolas. 1977. *The incubus in English literature: Provenance and progeny.* Pullman, WA: Washington State University Press.

Kingston, Maxine Hong. 1989. *The woman warrior: Memoirs of a girlhood among ghosts.* New York, NY: Vintage.

Kirschner, Robert H., Friedrich A. Eckner, and Roy C. Baron. 1986. The cardiac pathology of sudden, unexplained nocturnal death in Southeast Asian refugees. *Journal of the American Medical Association* 256(19): 2700–2705.

Kittredge, George Lyman. 1956. *Witchcraft in old and new England.* New York: Russell & Russell.

Klass, Perri. 1988. *UFO abductions: A dangerous game.* Buffalo, NY: Prometheus Books.

Kolb, Stephane, and Samuel Law. 2001. *Inuit perspectives on the 20th century: Dreams and dream interpretations.* Iqlauit, Nunavut: Nunavut Arctic College.

Kompanje, E. J. O. 2008. "The devil lay upon her and held her down": Hypnagogic hallucinations and sleep paralysis described by the Dutch physician Isbrand Van Diemerbroeck (1609–1674) in 1664. *Journal of Sleep Research* 17(4): 464–467.

Kotorii, T., T. Kotorii, N. Uchimura, Y. Hashizume, S. Shirakawa, T. Satomura, J. Tanaka, et al. 2001. Questionnaire relating to sleep paralysis. *Psychiatry and Clinical Neurosciences* 55(3): 265–266.

Kramer, Heinrich, and Jacob Sprenger. 1971. *Malleus maleficarum.* Trans. M. Summers. New York: Dover Publications. (Orig. pub. 1487.)

Kristoff, Nicholas D. 1999. "Alien abduction? Science calls it sleep paralysis." *New York Times,* 6 July, F1–8.

Krittayaphong, R, G. Veerakul, K. Nademanee, and C. Kangkagate. 2003. Heart rate variability in patients with Brugada syndrome in Thailand. *European Heart Journal* 24(19): 1771–1778.

Kryger, M. H., T. Roth, and W. C. Dement, eds. 2000. *Principles and practice of sleep medicine.* Philadelphia: W. B. Saunders.

Kuhn, Adalbert. 1859. *Sagen, Gebräuche, und Märchen aus Westfalen.* Leipzig: F. A. Brodhaus.

Laistner, Ludwig. 1889. *Das Rätsel der Sphinx. Grundzüge einer Mythengeschichte.* Berlin: W. Hertz.

Lars, Eckardt. 2007. Gender differences in Brugada syndrome. *Journal of Cardiovascular Electrophysiology* 18(4): 422–424.

Larteguy, Jean. 1979. *La fabuleuse aventure de peuple de l'opium*. Paris: Presses de la Cite.

Law, S., and L. J. Kirmayer. 2005. Inuit interpretations of sleep paralysis. *Transcultural Psychiatry* 42(1): 93–112.

Lecouteux, Claude. 1987. Mara-ephialtes-incubus: Le cauchemar chez les peuples Germaniques. *Etudes Germaniques* 42: 1–24.

Lee, Gary Yia. 1994–95. The religious presentation of social relationships: Hmong world view and social structure. *Lao Studies Review* 2: 44–60.

Lee, Mai Na M. 1998. Book review: *The spirit catches you and you fall down*. http://www.hmongnet.org/publications/spirit_review.html

Lemoine, Jacques. 1986. Shamanism in the context of Hmong resettlement. In *The Hmong in transition*, eds. G. L. Hendricks, B. T. Downing and A. S. Deinard, 337–348. Staten Island, NY: Center for Migration Studies of New York.

Lemoine, Jacques, and Christine Mougne. 1983. Why has death stalked the refugees? *Natural History* 92(11): 12–19.

Levin, Max. 1957. Premature waking and post-dormitial paralysis. *The Journal of Nervous and Mental Disease* 125(1): 140–142.

Levin, Max. 1961. Sleep, cataplexy, and fatigue as manifestations of Pavlovian inhibition. *American Journal of Psychotherapy* 15: 122–137.

Levin, Max. 1967. Sleep paralysis. *Current Medical Digest* 34: 1229, 1232.

Lewis, G. 1987. Fear of sorcery and the problem of death by suggestion. *Social Science and Medicine* 24(12): 997–1010.

Liddon, S. C. 1967. Sleep paralysis and hypnagogic hallucinations: Their relationship to the nightmare. *Archives of General Psychiatry* 17(1): 88–96.

Liddon, S. C. 1970. Sleep paralysis, psychosis, and death. *American Journal of Psychiatry* 126(7): 1027–1031.

Lifetime Network. 2007. *Nightmare*. Directed by Terry Ingram.

London, Barry, Michael Michalec, Haider Mehdi, Xiaodong Zhu, Laurie Kerchner, Shamarendra Sanyal, Prakash C. Viswanathan, et al. 2007. Mutation in glycerol-3-phosphate dehydrogenase 1-like gene (GPD1-L) decreases cardiac Na+ current and causes inherited arrhythmias. *Circulation* 116(20): 2260–2268.

Lovecraft, H. P. 1927. Supernatural horror in literature. *The Recluse* 1: 23–59.

Lown, B., J. V. Temte, P. Reich, C. Gaughan, Q. Regestein, and H. Hal. 1976. Basis for recurring ventricular fibrillation in the absence of coronary heart disease and its management. *New England Journal of Medicine* 294(12): 623–629.

Lown, B., and R. L. Verrier. 1976. Neural activity and ventricular fibrillation. *New England Journal of Medicine* 294(21): 1165–1170.

Luparello, T. J., N. Leist, C. H. Lourie, and P. Sweet. 1970. The interaction of psychologic stimuli and pharmacologic agents on airway reactivity in asthmatic subjects. *Psychosomatic Medicine* 32(5): 509–513.

Luparello, T. J., H. A. Lyons, E. R. Bleecker, and E. R. McFadden, Jr. 1968. Influences of suggestion on airway reactivity in asthmatic subjects. *Psychosomatic Medicine* 30(6): 819–825.

Mack, John E. 1994. *Abduction: Human encounters with aliens*. New York: Ballantine Books.

MacNish, Robert. 1834. *The philosophy of sleep*. New York: Appleton and Co.

Mandhur, Ibn. 2006. "Al-Jathum." In *Lisan al Arab: Dar kotob al ilmiyah*. eds. Amir Ahmad Haider and Abdul Munim Ibrahim. Lebanon: Dar al-Kutub al-Ilmiyah.

Marshall, Eliot. 1981. The Hmong: Dying of culture shock? *Science* 212(4498): 1008.

Marx, Karl. 1907. The eighteenth Brumaire of Louis Bonaparte. Trans. D. De Leon. Chicago: Charles H. Kerr & Co. (Orig. pub. 1852.)

Mather, Cotton. 1692. *Wonders of the invisible world.* New York: Dorset Press.

Matsuo, K., T. Kurita, M. Inagaki, M. Kakishita, N. Aihara, W. Shimizu, A. Taguchi, et al. 1999. The circadian pattern of the development of ventricular fibrillation in patients with Brugada syndrome. *European Heart Journal* 20(6): 465–470.

Maupassant, Guy de. 2007. *The Horla and Other Stories.* Trans. A.M.C. McMaster et al. New York: Wildside Press. (Orig. pub. 1887)

Mavromatis, Andreas. 1987. *Hypnagogia: The unique state of consciousness between wakefulness and sleep.* London: Routledge & Kegan Paul.

Maxwell, Evan. 1981a. "Mysterious fatal malady striking Hmong men." *Los Angeles Times,* 14 July, C1.

Maxwell, Evan. 1981b. "Refugees' medical mystery." *Los Angeles Times,* 12 July, OC-B1.

McNally, R. J., and S. A. Clancy. 2005. Sleep paralysis in adults reporting repressed, recovered, or continuous memories of childhood sexual abuse. *Journal of Anxiety Disorders* 19(5): 595–602.

McNamara, Patrick. 2008. *Nightmares.* Westport, CT and London: Praeger.

Mdlalani, Angela. 2009. "A sleep disorder worse than a nightmare." *Sunday Standard,* 13 December. http://www.sundaystandard.info/article.php?NewsID=6543&GroupID=2

Meier, Peg. 2004. "Unraveling a mystery." *Star Tribune,* 21 August, E1.

Mellman, Thomas A, Notalelomwan Aigbogun, Ruth Elaine Graves, William B. Lawson, and Tanya N. Alim. 2008. Sleep paralysis and trauma, psychiatric symptoms and disorders in an adult African American population attending primary medical care. *Depression and Anxiety* 25(5): 435–440.

Melville, Herman. 1851. *Moby-dick; or, the whale.* New York: Harper and Brothers.

Meredith, William H., and George P. Rowe. 1986. Changes in Hmong refugee marital attitudes in America. In *The Hmong in transition,* eds. G. L. Hendricks, B. T. Downing, and A. S. Deinard, 121–133. Staten Island, NY: Center for Migration Studies of New York.

Miller, Steve. 2005. "Racial abuse linked to hunter shooting." *Washington Times,* 30 January. http://www.washingtontimes.com/news/2005/jan/30/20050130-123456-1371r/

Milton, Gerald W. 1973. Self-willed death or the bone-pointing syndrome. *The Lancet* 1(7817): 1435–1436.

Mishler, Elliot G., Lorna R. Amarasingham, Samuel D. Osherson, Stuart t. Hauser, Nancy E. Waxler, and Ramsay Liem. 1981. *Social Contexts of Health, Illness, and Patient Care.* New York and Cambridge: Cambridge University Press.

Mitchell, Silas Weir. 1876. Some disorders of sleep. *Virginia Medical Monthly* 2: 769–781.

Miura, D., K. Nakamura, and T. Ohe. 2008. Update on genetic analysis in Brugada syndrome. *Heart Rhythm* 5(10): 1495–1496.

Moerman, Daniel E. 2002. *Meaning, medicine, and the "placebo effect."* Cambridge: Cambridge University Press.

Montagu-Nathan, N. 1917. Promenade concerts. *Musical Times* 58(895): 417–418.

Moody, Raymond A. 1975. *Life after life: The investigation of a phenomenon—survival of bodily death.* Atlanta, GA: Mockingbird Books.

Morin, Stephen P. 1983. "Troubled refugees: Many Hmong, puzzled by life in U.S., yearn for old days in Laos." *Wall Street Journal,* 16 February, 1.

Morris, David B. 2000. *Illness and culture in the postmodern age.* Berkeley, CA: University of California Press.

Morrow, Gary R., and Patricia L. Dobkin. 1988. Anticipatory nausea and vomiting in cancer patients undergoing chemotherapy treatment: Prevalence, etiology, and behavioral interventions. *Clinical Psychology Review* 8(5): 517–556.

Mortazavi, S. M., J. Ahmadi, and M. Shariati. 2007. Prevalence of subjective poor health symptoms associated with exposure to electromagnetic fields among university students. *Bioelectromagnetics* 28(4): 326–330.

Moturi, Sricharan, and Anna Ivanenko. 2009. Complex diagnostic and treatment issues in psychotic symptoms associated with narcolepsy. *Psychiatry* 6(6): 38–44.

Munger, Ronald G., and Marshall G. Hurlich. 1981. Hmong deaths. *Science* 213(4511): 952.

Mydans, Seth. 1990. "California says Laos refugee group is a victim of leadership's extortion." *New York Times,* 7 November, A20.

Nelson, K. R., M. Mattingly, and F. A. Schmitt. 2007. Out-of-body experience and arousal. *Neurology* 68(10): 794–795.

Ness, Robert C. 1978. The old hag phenomenon as sleep paralysis: A biocultural interpretation. *Culture, Medicine, and Psychiatry* 2(1): 15–39.

Newman, L. S., and R. F. Baumeister. 1996. Toward an explanation of the UFO abduction phenomenon: Hypnotic elaboration, extraterrestrial sadomasochism, and spurious memories. *Psychological Inquiry* 7(2): 99–126.

Oftedal, G., A. Straume, A. Johnsson, and L. J. Stovner. 2007. Mobile phone headache: A double blind, sham-controlled provocation study. *Cephalalgia* 27(5): 447–455.

Ohaeri, J. U. 1992. Experience of isolated sleep paralysis in clinical practice in Nigeria. *Journal of the National Medical Association* 84(6): 521–523.

Ohayon, M. M., J. Zulley, C. Guilleminault, and S. Smirne. 1999. Prevalence and pathologic associations of sleep paralysis in the general population. *Neurology* 52(6): 1194–1200.

Ong, Aihwa. 2003. *Buddha is hiding: Refugees, citizenship, the new America.* Berkeley, CA: University of California Press.

Otto, C. M., R. V. Tauxe, L. A. Cobb, H. L. Greene, B. W. Gross, J. A. Werner, R. W. Burroughs, et al. 1984. Ventricular fibrillation causes sudden death in Southeast Asian immigrants. *Annals of Internal Medicine* 101(1): 45–47.

Otto, Rudolf. 1926. *The idea of the holy.* Trans. J. W. Harvey. London: Oxford Press.

The Oxford English Dictionary. 1989. J. A. Simpson and E. S. C. Weiner, eds. 2nd ed. Oxford: Clarendon Press.

Paradis, C. M., and S. Friedman. 2005. Sleep paralysis in African Americans with panic disorder. *Transcultural Psychiatry* 42(1): 123–134.

Paradis, C. M., S. Friedman, and M. Hatch. 1997. Isolated sleep paralysis in African Americans with panic disorder. *Cultural Diversity and Mental Health* 3(1): 69–76.

Parkes, C. M., B. Benjamin, and R. G. Fitzgerald. 1969. Broken heart: A statistical study of increased mortality among widowers. *British Medical Journal* 1(646): 740–743.

Parrish, Roy Gibson. 1988. Death in the night: Mysterious syndrome in Asian refugees. In *1989 medical and health annual,* eds. E. Bernstein and L. Tomchuck. Chicago: Encyclopedia Britannica.

Parrish, Roy Gibson, Myra Tucker, Roy Ing, Carol Encarnacion, and Mark Eberhardt. 1987. Sudden unexplained death syndrome in Southeast Asian refugees: A review of CDC surveillance. *Morbidity and Mortality Weekly Report (MMWR) CDC Surveillance Summaries* 36(1): 43–53.

Patai, Raphael. 1990. *The Hebrew goddess,* 3rd ed. Detroit, MI: Wayne State University Press.

Payn, S. B. 1965. A psychoanalytic approach to sleep paralysis. Review and report of a case. *Journal of Nervous and Mental Disease* 140(6): 427–433.

Pearce, J. M. 1993. Early descriptions of sleep paralysis. *Journal of Neurology, Neurosurgery, and Psychiatry* 56(12): 1302.

Pendergrast, M. 1996. *Victims of memory: Sex abuse accusations and shattered lives.* London: HarperCollins.

Peterson, Sally. 1988. Translating experience and the reading of a story cloth. *Journal of American Folklore* 101(399): 6–22.

Phillips, D. P., T. E. Ruth, and L. M. Wagner. 1993. Psychology and survival. *The Lancet* 342(8880): 1142–1145.

Poe, Edgar Allan. 1845. *Tales.* New York: Wiley and Putnam.

Powell, Nicolas. 1973. *Fuseli: The nightmare.* New York: Viking Press.

Proud, Louis. 2009. *Dark intrusions: An investigation into the paranormal nature of sleep paralysis experiences.* San Antonio, TX, and New York: Anomalist Books.

Pyle, Jack. 1981. "Death stalking refugees." *News Tribune* (Tacoma, Washington), 16 April., C1.

Quincy, Keith. 1995. *Hmong, history of a people,* 2nd ed. Cheney, WA: Eastern Washington University.

Randle, K.D., R. Estes, and W. P. Cone. 1999. *The abduction enigma: The truth behind the mass alien abductions of the late twentieth century.* New York: Forge.

Rawlinson, Henry Creswicke. 1861–1864. *The cuneiform inscriptions of Western Asia.* 5 vols. London: Trustees of the British Museum.

Rechtschaffen, Allan, and William C. Dement. 1969. Narcolepsy and hypersomnia. In *Sleep: Physiology & pathology; a symposium,* ed. A. Kales, 119–130. Philadelphia: Lippincott.

Reich, P., R. A. DeSilva, B. Lown, and B. J. Murawski. 1981. Acute psychological disturbances preceding life-threatening ventricular arrhythmias. *Journal of the American Medical Association* 246(3): 233–235.

Reid, Brian. 2002. "The nocebo effect: Placebo's evil twin." *The Washington Post,* 30 April, HE01.

Reid, Janice, and Nancy Williams. 1984. "Voodoo death" in Arnhem Land: Whose reality? *American Anthropologist* 86(1): 121–133.

Revill, Jo. 2006. "Sleep—our new obsession." *The Observer,* 9 April, 23.

Richter, C. P. 1957. On the phenomenon of sudden death in animals and man. *Psychosomatic Medicine* 19(3): 191–198.

Rickels, Patricia K. 1961. Some accounts of witch riding. *Louisiana Folklore Miscellany* 2(1): 53–63.

Roberts, Katherine. 1998. Contemporary cauchemar: Experience, belief, prevention. *Louisiana Folklore Miscellany* 13: 15–26.

Rønnevig, Georg M. 2007. Toward an explanation of the "abduction epidemic": The ritualization of alien abduction mythology in therapeutic settings. In *Alien worlds: Social and religious dimensions of extraterrestrial contact,* ed. D. G. Tumminia, 99–127. Syracuse, NY: Syracuse University Press.

Roscher, Wilhelm Heinrich. 1900. *Pan and the nightmare: Being the only English translation (from the German by A. V. O'Brien) of Ephialtes, a pathological-mythological treatise on the nightmare in classical antiquity.* Irving, TX: Spring Publications.

Rowley, Jason T., Robert Stickgold, and J. Allan Hobson. 1988. Eyelid movements and mental activity at sleep onset. *Consciousness and Cognition* 7(1): 67–84.

Rushton, J. G. 1944. Sleep paralysis. *Medical Clinics of North America* 28: 945–949.

Sandstrom, M., J. Wilen, G. Oftedal, and K. Hansson Mild. 2001. Mobile phone use and subjective symptoms: Comparison of symptoms experienced by users of analogue and digital mobile phones. *Occupational Medicine* 51(1): 25–35.

Savina, F. M. 1924. *Histoire des Miao.* Hong Kong: Societe des Missions Etrangeres de Paris.

Sayce, A. H. 1900. Cairene folklore. *Folk-Lore* 2(4): 387.

Scerba, Amy 1999. Changing literary representations of Lilith and the evolution of a mythical heroine. M.A. thesis, Carnegie Mellon University.

Schacter, D. L. 1976. The hypnagogic state: A critical review of the literature. *Psychological Bulletin* 83(3): 452–481.

Schegoleva, Anna. 2002. Sleepless in Japan: The kanashibari phenomenon. Paper presented at the proceedings of a postgraduate research seminar in Japanese studies at Oxford Brookes University Research Centre, Oxford, UK.

Schenck, Carlos H. 2007. *Sleep: A groundbreaking guide to the mysteries, the problems, and the solutions*. New York: Avery.

Scheper-Hughes, Nancy, and Margaret M. Lock. 1987. The mindful body: A prolegomenon to future work in medical anthropology. *Medical Anthropology Quarterly*, New Series, 1(1): 6–41.

Schiffman, Aldona Christina. 1987. The witch and crime: The persecution of witches in twentieth-century Poland. *ARV: Scandinavian Yearbook of Folklore* 43: 147–165.

Schneck, J. M. 1948. Sleep paralysis: Psychodynamics. *Psychiatric Quarterly* 22(3): 462–469.

Schneck, J. M. 1957. Sleep paralysis: A new evaluation. *Diseases of the Nervous System* 18(4): 144–146.

Schonberger, Stephen. 1946. A clinical contribution to the analysis of the nightmare-syndrome. *Psychoanalytic Review* 33: 44–70.

ScienceDaily. 2007. Cardiologists identify new cardiac arrest gene. *ScienceDaily*, http://www.sciencedaily.com /releases/2007/10/071031114325.htm

Scot, Reginald. 1584. *Discoverie of witchcraft*. London: Richard Cotes.

Sevilla, Jorge Conesa. 2004. *Wresting with ghosts: A personal and scientific account of sleep paralysis*. Philadelphia: Xlibris.

Shakespeare, William. 2004. *Romeo and Juliet*. New York: Simon and Schuster. (Orig. pub. 1623.)

Shelley, Mary Wollstonecraft. 1831. *Frankenstein; or, the modern Prometheus*. London: Henry Colburn and Richard Bentley.

Sherman, Spencer. 1988. The Hmong in America: Laotian refugees in "the land of the giants." *National Geographic* 174(4): 586–610.

Sherwood, Simon J. 2002. Relationship between the hypnagogic/hypnopompic states and reports of anomalous experiences. *Journal of Parapsychology* 66(2): 127–150.

Shulins, Nancy. 1984. "Hmong refugees undergo severe culture shock." *Los Angeles Times*, 8 July, 2.

Simpson, Alan. 1987. Quoted in "Senate holds midyear hearings on FY87 refugee admissions." *Refugee Reports* 8(July): 4.

Skinner, Margot A., Ruth N. Kingshott, Sue Filsell, and D. Robin Taylor. 2008. Efficacy of the "tennis ball technique" versus Ncpap in the management of position-dependent obstructive sleep apnoea syndrome. *Respirology* 13(5). 708–715.

Sleep Paralysis Information Service. 2009. *How to avoid an episode of sleep paralysis*, http://www.spis.org.uk

Snyder, S. 1983. ISP after rapid time-zone change ("jet-lag") syndrome. *Chronobiologia* 10: 377–379.

Spalding, Thomas. 1880. *Elizabethan demonology*. London: Chatto and Windus.

Spanos, Nicholas P. 1996. *Multiple identities and false memories: A sociocognitive perspective*. Washington, DC: American Psychological Association.

Spanos, Nicholas P., Patricia A. Cross, Kirby Dickson, and Susan C. DuBreuil. 1993. Close encounters: An examination of UFO experiences. *Journal of Abnormal Psychology* 102(4): 624–632.

Spanos, Nicholas P., Stacey A. McNulty, Susan C. DuBreuil, Martha Pires, and Melissa Faith Burgess. 1995. The frequency and correlates of sleep paralysis in a university sample. *Journal of Research in Personality* 29(3): 285–305.

Spiegel, H. 1997. Nocebo: The power of suggestibility. *Preventive Medicine* 26(5 Pt 1): 616–621.

Steiner, Rudolf. 1999. The dead are always with us. In *Staying connected: How to continue your relationships with those who have died,* 141–161. Great Barrington, MA: Anthroposophic Press.

Steger, Brigitte, and Lodewijk Brunt, eds. 2003. *Night-time and sleep in Asia and the West: Exploring the dark side of life.* New York and London: Routledge.

Stern, David, and Mark Jay Mirsky, eds. 1998. *Rabbinic fantasies: Imaginative narratives from classical Hebrew literature.* New Haven, CT: Yale University Press.

Sternberg, Esther M. 2002. Walter B. Cannon and "voodoo' death": A perspective from 60 years on. *American Journal of Public Health* 92(10): 1564–1566.

Stevenson, Robert Louis. 1886. *Kidnapped.* London: Cassell.

Stewart, Charles. 2002. Erotic dreams and nightmares from antiquity to the present. *Journal of the Royal Anthropological Institute* 8(2): 279–309.

Stol, Marten. 1993. *Epilepsy in Babylonia.* Groningen, The Netherlands: Brill Academic Publishers.

Stores, G. 1998. Sleep paralysis and hallucinosis. *Behavioral Neurology* 11(2): 109–112.

Stovner, L. J., G. Oftedal, A. Straume, and A. Johnsson. 2008. Nocebo as headache trigger: Evidence from a sham-controlled provocation study with RF fields. *Acta Neurologica Scandinavica* 117(188): 67–71.

Sturluson, Snorri. 1932. *Heimskringla; or, the lives of the Norse kings.* Trans. A. H. Smith. Cambridge: W. Heffer & Sons.

Taitt, Paul, and Andrew Barnes. 2008. *Your worst nightmare: Supernatural assault.* DVD. Soul Smack Production.

Takahashi, Yumi. 2009. *Pokkuri-dera: The meaning of longevity among Japanese elderly,* http://homepages.wmich.edu/~weinreic/GRN670/Japan/PokurriDerai.html

Takeuchi, T., A. Miyasita, Y. Sasaki, M. Inugami, and K. Fukuda. 1992. Isolated sleep paralysis elicited by sleep interruption. *Sleep* 15(3): 217–225.

Terrillon, Jean-Christophe, and Sirley Marques-Bonham. 2001. Does recurrent isolated sleep paralysis involve more than cognitive neurosciences? *Journal of Scientific Exploration* 15(1): 97–123.

Thao, Xoua. 1986. Hmong perception of illness and traditional ways of healing. In *The Hmong in transition,* eds. G. L. Hendricks, B. T. Downing and A. S. Deinard. Staten Island, NY: Center for Migration Studies of New York.

Thatcher, James. 1826. *American modern practice.* Boston: Cottons and Barnard.

Thomas, Ronald R. 1992. *Dreams of authority: Freud and the fictions of the unconscious.* Ithaca, NY: Cornell University Press.

Thompson, M. 1986. The Elusive Promise. *Far Eastern Economic Review* 134: 46–49.

Thompson, R. Campbell. 1903. *The devils and evil spirits of Babylonia.* Vol. 1. London: Luzac and Co.

Thompson, R. Campbell. 1908. *Semitic magic: Its origins and development.* London: Luzac and Co.

Thompson, Stith. 1955. *Motif-index of folk-literature; a classification of narrative elements in folktales, ballads, myths, fables, mediaeval romances, exempla, fabliaux, jest-books, and local legends.* Rev. and enl. ed. Bloomington, IN: Indiana University Press.

Tillhagen, C. H. 1969. The conception of the nightmare in Sweden. In *Humaniora,* eds. W. D. Hand and G. O. Arlt. New York: Augustin.

Tobin, J. J., and J. Friedman. 1983. Spirits, shamans, and nightmare death: Survivor stress in a Hmong refugee. *American Journal of Orthopsychiatry* 53(3): 439–448.

Todd, Janet. 2000. *Mary Wollstonecraft: A revolutionary life*. London: Weidenfeld and Nicolson.

Traphgan, J. W. 2000. *Taming oblivion: Aging bodies and the fear of senility in Japan*. Albany, NY: State University of New York Press.

Uhde, Thomas W., Bernadette M. Cortese, and Andrei Vedeniapin. 2009. Anxiety and sleep problems: Emerging concepts and theoretical treatment implications. *Current Psychiatry Reports* 11(4): 269–276.

Uhde, Thomas W., Orlena Merritt-Davis, and Yuri Yaroslavsky. 2006. Sleep paralysis: Overlooked fearful arousal. Abstract 96D. *Proceedings of the 159th Annual Meeting of the American Psychiatric Association*. Washington, DC: American Psychiatric Association.

Ulrich, R. S. 1984. View through a window may influence recovery from surgery. *Science* 224(4647): 420–421.

University of Kentucky. 2007. Out-of-body experiences may be caused by arousal system disturbances in brain. *ScienceDaily*, 6 March, http://www.sciencedaily.com/releases/2007/03/070305202657.htm

Van Der Heide, Carel, and Jack Weinberg. 1945. Sleep paralysis and combat fatigue. *Psychosomatic Medicine* 7(6): 330–334.

Van Diemerbroeck, Isband. 1664. *Disputationum practicarum pars prima & secunda, de morbis capitis & thoracis*. Utrecht: Th. van Ackerdyck.

Van Dongen, Hans P. A., Greg Maislin, Janet M. Mullington, and David F. Dinges. 2003. The cumulative cost of additional wakefulness: Dose-response effects on neurobehavioral functions and sleep physiology from chronic sleep restriction and total sleep deprivation. *Sleep* 26(2): 117–126.

Vang, Lo. 1987. Letter to Senator Alan Simpson. (29 July). Southeast Asia Resource Action Center records, Special Collections and Archives, UC Irvine Libraries.

Vang, Lue, and Lewis, Judy. 1984. *Grandmother's Path, Grandfather's Way*. Rancho Cordova, California: Zellerbach Family Fund.

Verdecchia, P., J. A. Staessen, W. B. White, Y. Imai, and E. T. O'Brien. 2002. Properly defining white coat hypertension. *European Heart Journal* 23(2): 106–109.

Vickers, Marcia. 1997. "After tripping on its laces, Reebok is focused again." *New York Times*, 2 March, 3.

Viviano, Frank. 1986. From the Asian hills to a U.S. valley. *Far Eastern Economic Review* 134: 47–49.

Waller, John Augustine. 1816. *A treatise on the incubus, or, nightmare, disturbed sleep, terrific dreams, and nocturnal visions; with the means of removing these distressing complaints*. London: Cox.

Walsh, Michael. 2009. The politicisation of Popobawa: Changing explanations of a collective panic in Zanzibar. *Journal of Humanities* 1(1): 23–33.

Ward, Donald J. 1977. The little man who wasn't there: Encounters with the supranormal. *Fabula: Journal of Folklore Studies* 18: 213–225.

Ward, Donald J. 1981. *The German legends of the brothers Grimm*. 2 vols. Trans. D. J. Ward. Philadelphia: Institute for the Study of Human Issues.

Ward, Maryanne C. 2000. A painting of the unspeakable: Henry Fuseli's "The Nightmare" and the creation of Mary Shelley's "Frankenstein." *Journal of the Midwest Modern Language Association* 33(1): 20–31.

Weinger, Matthew B., and Sonia Ancoli-Israel. 2002. Sleep deprivation and clinical performance. *Journal of the American Medical Association* 287(8): 955–957.

Westermeyer, J. 1981. Hmong deaths. *Science* 213: 952.

Westermeyer, J. 1987. Prevention of mental disorder among Hmong refugees in the U.S.: Lessons from the period 1976–1986. *Social Science and Medicine* 25(8): 941–947.

Westermeyer, J. 1988. A matched pairs study of depression among Hmong refugees with particular reference to predisposing factors and treatment outcome. *Social Psychiatry and Psychiatric Epidemiology* 23(1): 64–71.

Weyer, Johann. 1563. *De praestigiis daemonum et incantationibus ac venificiis.* Basel, Switzerland: J. Oporinum.

Whitaker, Elizabeth D., ed. 2006. *Health and healing in comparative perspective.* Upper Saddle River, NJ: Pearson Prentice-Hall.

Whitman, David. 1987. Trouble for America's "Model Minority." U.S. News and World Report February 23: 18–19.

Wichter, T., E. Schulze-Bahr, M. Paul, G. Breithardt, and L. Eckardt. 2006. Drug Challenge in Brugada Syndrome: How Valuable is It? In *Cardiac arrhythmias 2005: Proceedings of the 9th International Workshop on Cardiac Arrhythmias,* ed. A. Raviele, 303–315. Italy: Springer.

Wilson, Colin. 2006. *Mysteries: An investigation into the occult, the paranormal, and the supernatural.* New York: Sterling Publishing Company.

Wilson, S. A. Kinnier. 1928. The narcolepsies. *Brain* 51(1): 63–109.

Wing, Y. K., H. Chiu, T. Leung, and J. Ng. 1999. Sleep paralysis in the elderly. *Journal of Sleep Research* 8(2): 151–155.

Wing, Y. K., S. T. Lee, and C. N. Chen. 1994. Sleep paralysis in Chinese: Ghost oppression phenomenon in Hong Kong. *Sleep* 17(7): 609–613.

Worthman, Carol M., and Melissa K. Melby. 2002. Toward a comparative developmental ecology of human sleep. In *Adolescent sleep patterns: Biological, social, and psychological influences,* ed. M. A. Carskadon, 69–117. New York: Cambridge University Press.

Wright, D. 1994. Initial findings of the abduction transcription project. *Mutual UFO Network (MUFON) Journal* 310/311: 3–7.

Wright, Lawrence. 1993. Remembering Satan (parts I and II). *The New Yorker,* 17 May, 60; 24 May, 54.

Wright, Lawrence. 1995. *Remembering Satan: A tragic case of recovered memory.* New York: Vintage.

Yang, D., and D. North. 1988. *Profiles of the highland Lao communities in the United States, final report,* ed. F. S. A. Office of Refugee Resettlement. Washington, DC: U.S. Dept. of Health and Human Services.

Yang, Yeng. 1998. Practicing modern medicine: "A little medicine, a little neeb." *Hmong Studies Journal* 2(2): 1–7.

INDEX

Page numbers in italics refer to illustrations.

ABOUT THE AUTHOR

SHELLEY R. ADLER, PhD, is a professor in the Department of Family and Community Medicine and the director of education at the Osher Center for Integrative Medicine at the University of California, San Francisco.